KETO DIET AFTER 50

THE ULTIMATE KETOGENIC DIET FOR MEN AND WOMEN OVER 50. BURN FAT, AND PREVENT DISEASES BY FIXING YOUR METABOLISM AND STAY HEALTHY EVEN IN YOUR SENIOR YEARS WITH 21-DAY MEAL PLAN

By

Paty Breads

TABLE OF CONTENTS

INTRODUCTION **4**

CHAPTER 1: HOW THE KETOGENIC DIET WORKS? **6**

CHAPTER 2: BENEFITS OF GOING ON A KETOGENIC DIET **9**

CHAPTER 3: HOW TO START A KETO DIET WHEN YOU'RE OVER 50? **16**

CHAPTER 4: HOW DOES AGING AFFECT YOUR NUTRITIONAL NEEDS **20**

CHAPTER 5: BENEFITS OF THE KETO DIET FOR PEOPLE OVER 50 ....**23**

CHAPTER 6: KETO SIDE EFFECTS AND HOW TO SALVE THEM **26**

CHAPTER 7: KETO GROCERY LIST **31**

CHAPTER 8: LET'S TALK ABOUT PRODUCTS **38**

    ALLOWED PRODUCT LIST 38

    PROHIBITED PRODUCT LIST 42

CHAPTER 9: EXERCISES TO ASSIST WITH QUALITY OF LIFE AFTER 50 ..**44**

CHAPTER 10: ADDITIONAL THINGS THAT CAN HELP **50**

CHAPTER 11: 21-DAY KETO MEAL PLAN **55**

CHAPTER 12: BREAKFAST RECIPES **57**

    CRISPY WAFFLES 57

    ANTI INFLAMMATORY MUFFINS 59

    MINI CRUSTLESS QUICHES...60

    FRENCH BAKED EGGS 62

    ZINGY SCRAMBLE 63

    NO-COOKING BREAKFAST BOWL 64

    SUPER FOOD SMOOTHIE BOWL 65

    NUTTY TEXTURED PORRIDGE..66

CHAPTER 13: LUNCH RECIPES **67**

    BACON BURGER CABBAGE STIR FRY 67

    BACON CHEESEBURGER...68

    CAULIFLOWER MAC & CHEESE 69

    MUSHROOM & CAULIFLOWER RISOTTO 70

    PITA PIZZA 71

    SKILLET CABBAGE TACOS..72

    TACO CASSEROLE..73

    CREAMY CHICKEN SALAD...74

    SPICY KETO CHICKEN WINGS 75

    CILANTRO AND LIME CREAMED CHICKEN 77

    CHEESY HAM QUICHE..78

Loaded Cauliflower Rice 79
Super Herbed Fish 80

CHAPTER 14: DINNER RECIPES **81**

Chicken Pan with Veggies and Pesto 81
Cabbage Soup with Beef 82
Cauliflower Rice Soup with Chicken 83
Quick Pumpkin Soup 85
Fresh Avocado Soup 86
Creamy Garlic Chicken 87
Cauliflower Cheesecake 88
Chinese Pork Bowl 89
Turkey-Pepper Mix 90
Shrimp Scampi with Garlic 91
Simple Tuna Salad 92

CHAPTER 15: VEGETABLES RECIPES **93**

Scrumptious Cauliflower Casserole 93
Relatively Flavored Gratin 95
Thanksgiving Veggie Meal 96
Loaded Squash Casserole 98
Meatless Cabbage Rolls 99

CHAPTER 16: DESSERTS RECIPES **101**

British Tartlets 101
Sweet & Tangy Tart 103
Flour less Chocolate Cake 105
Melt-in-Moth Lava Cake 106
British Tartlets 107
Sweet & Tangy Tart 108
Light Greek Yogurt Cheesecake 110
Swiss Roll Cake 111

CHAPTER 17: SNACKS RECIPES **113**

Crispy Broccoli Pop Corn 113
Cheesy Cauliflower Croquettes 115
Spinach in Cheese Envelopes 116
Cheesy Mushroom Slices 117
Kale Chips 119
Guacamole 120
Zucchini Noodles 121
Cauliflower Souffle 122

CHAPTER 18: TIPS ON LOSING WEIGHT ON KETO AFTER 50 ....**123**

CONCLUSION **131**

Introduction

Keto diet is a diet plan that consists of low-carb and high-fat food items which directly forces our body to burn all the fat for body energy in place of sugar and carbs. The keto diet forces our body to use up the stored fat which allows the fat cells of the body to release all the fatty acids. The fatty acids, in turn, get converted into ketones by the liver. As soon as this process starts, the body gets into the state of ketosis, where ketones are burnt down for energy instead of sugar or glucose. As the overall intake of carbs gets reduced in this form of the diet, the ketones turn out to be the main energy source. This ultimately results in a significant amount of weight loss.

A Ketogenic Diet is something that you should be starting off with today for a better lifestyle if you are over the age of 50. The ketogenic diet is more common in women than in men because of all the benefits that it provides for dealing with the symptoms of menopause. Women who are experiencing menopause, or have already experienced it, have a clear idea of the troubles that come along with it. Menopause leads to fatigue, irritability, and also increases weight. But the keto diet can really help in controlling your body weight and also improve your physical well-being. Not sure from where or how to start with keto?

As the diet continues to grow in popularity, there is more research being performed on the Ketogenic Diet by the day! With science-backed evidence, you can follow the diet and know for a fact that it is going to work.

Welcome to your first Ketogenic Diet Science lesson! One of the best parts of the Ketogenic Diet is the fact that it is based around a natural process that your body already has! The key to success is fueling your body correctly instead of stuffing it with overly-processed junk. In this guide, you will learn everything you need to know from what to eat when to eat and how to get into the best shape of your life!

The first lesson you need to know is that our body has four primary fuels that we use. These include glucose, protein, free fatty acids, and ketones. Each one of these fuel sources are stored in different proportions in our bodies. Overall, the fuel that we use the most is stored as triglyceride in our adipose tissue, aka, FAT! The second most used source is protein and glucose, which are used depending upon the metabolic state of your body.

So, what determines what fuel to use and when? As you might have already guessed, the primary determinant is based upon carbohydrate availability. Additional factors that can affect fuel utilization include a full or empty liver glycogen level and the levels of certain enzymes. Overall, total energy equals glucose plus FFA.

Next, it is vital that you understand that the body has three different fuel storages that it taps into when you begin to lower your calories. These three different storage depots include protein, carbohydrates, and fats! Protein is essential in your diet because it can be converted into glucose in your liver and then used as energy. Carbohydrates are typically stored as glycogen and are placed in your liver and muscle. Fat, on the other hand, is generally stored as body fat, but we will get to that in a second.

When you are following a SAD diet or a Standard American Diet, ketones truly have a non-existent role when it comes to your energy production. However, as you begin a ketogenic diet, it will play a much more significant role, and here we introduce the fourth potential fuel source for your body! As you start to decrease the carbohydrate availability through diet, your body will automatically make the shift to using fat as your first fuel source.

Chapter 1:

How the Ketogenic Diet Works?

What Happens to Your Body When You Eat Keto?

Even before we talk about how to do keto – it's important to first consider why this particular diet works. What actually happens to your body to make you lose weight?

As you probably know, the body uses food as an energy source. Everything you eat is turned into energy, so that you can get up and do whatever you need to accomplish for the day. The main energy source is sugar so what happens is that you eat something, the body breaks it down into sugar, and the sugar is processed into energy. Typically, the "sugar" is taken directly from the food you eat so if you eat just the right amount of food, then your body is fueled for the whole day. If you eat too much, then the sugar is stored in your body – hence the accumulation of fat.

But what happens if you eat less food? This is where the Ketogenic Diet comes in. You see, the process of creating sugar from food is usually faster if the food happens to be rich in carbohydrates. Bread, rice, grain, pasta – all of these are carbohydrates and they're the easiest food types to turn into energy.

So the Ketogenic Diet is all about reducing the amount of carbohydrates you eat. Does this mean you won't get the kind of energy you need for the day? Of course not! It only means that now, your body has to find other possible sources of energy. Do you know where they will be getting that energy? Your stored body fat!

So here's the situation – you are eating less carbohydrates every day. To keep you energetic, the body breaks down the stored fat and turns them into molecules called ketone bodies. The process of turning the fat into ketone bodies is called "Ketosis" and obviously – this is where the name of the Ketogenic Diet comes from. The ketone bodies take the place of glucose in keeping you energetic. As long as you keep your carbohydrates reduced, the body will keep getting its energy from your body fat.

Sounds Simple, Right?

The Ketogenic Diet is often praised for its simplicity and when you look at it properly, the process is really straightforward. The Science behind the effectivity of the diet is also well-documented, and has been proven multiple times by different medical fields. For example, an article on Diet Review by Harvard provided a lengthy discussion on how the Ketogenic Diet works and why it is so effective for those who choose to use this diet.

But Fat Is the Enemy…Or Is It?

No – fat is NOT the enemy. Unfortunately, years of bad science told us that fat is something you have to avoid – but it's actually a very helpful thing for weight loss! Even before we move forward with this book, we'll have to discuss exactly what "healthy fats" are, and why they're actually the good guys. To do this, we need to make a distinction between the different kinds of fat. You've probably heard of them before and it is a little bit confusing at first. We'll try to go through them as simply as possible:

Saturated fat. This is the kind you want to avoid. They're also called "solid fat" because each molecule is packed with hydrogen atoms. Simply put, it's the kind of fat that can easily cause a blockage in your body. It can raise cholesterol levels and lead to heart problems or a stroke. Saturated fat is something you can find in meat, dairy products, and other processed food items. Now, you're probably wondering: isn't the Ketogenic Diet packed with saturated fat? The answer is: not necessarily. You'll find later in the recipes given that the Ketogenic Diet promotes primarily unsaturated fat or healthy fat. While there are definitely many meat recipes in the list, most of these recipes contain healthy fat sources.

Unsaturated Fat. These are the ones dubbed as healthy fat. They're the kind of fat you find in avocado, nuts, and other ingredients you usually find in Keto-friendly recipes. They're known to lower blood cholesterol and actually come in two types: polyunsaturated and monounsaturated. Both are good for your body but the benefits slightly vary, depending on what you're consuming.

Polyunsaturated fat. These are perhaps the best in the list. You know about omega-3 fatty acids right? They're often suggested for people who have heart problems and are recognized as the "healthy" kind of fat. Well, they fall under the category of polyunsaturated fat and are known for reducing risks of heart disease by as much as 19 percent. This is according to a study titled: Effects on coronary heart diseases of increased poly-unsaturated fat in lieu of saturated fat: systematic review & meta-analysis of randomized controlled tests. So where do you get these polyunsaturated fats? You can get them mostly from vegetable and seed oils. These are ingredients you can almost always find in Ketogenic Recipes such as olive oil, coconut oil, and more. If you need more convincing, you should also know that omega-3 fatty acids are actually a kind of polyunsaturated fats and you will find them in deep sea fish like tuna, herring, and salmon.

Chapter 2:

Benefits Of Going On A Ketogenic Diet

As you can tell, there are some extremely complex biological processes behind the Ketogenic Diet. When you first start this diet out, you will want to consult with a doctor before you begin any changes. As far as any diet goes, it is crucial that you choose one that is going to benefit you rather than do more harm. For this reason, be sure to consult with a professional before you experiment on yourself.

With that in mind, why begin any diet if it isn't going to benefit you? Before you dive into the diet itself, let's learn all of the incredible ways that the Ketogenic Diet can help you. Whether you are looking to lose weight, gain energy, or improve brain function, the ketogenic diet may be just what you were searching for.

<u>Brain Benefits</u>

As you begin to change the fuel source for your body, this includes significant fuel sources for your brain as well. Studies have found that through the Ketogenic Diet, individuals were able to increase the stability of their neurons as well as the up-regulation of the mitochondrial enzymes and brain mitochondria.

With that in mind, scientists have been studying how a Ketogenic Diet may be able to benefit those who have Alzheimer's disease. It seems as though through diet, individuals have been able to enhance their memory as well as increase cognition. When this happens, a diet may be able to bring improvement to individuals with all different stages of dementia.

For those who do not need to worry about Parkinson's disease or Alzheimer's Disease, the Ketogenic Diet is also beneficial in increasing mental focus, clarity, and could potentially grant less frequent and less intense migraines. Generally, these conditions are related to altered brain chemistry and stable blood sugar levels, both helped by the Ketogenic Diet.

<u>Heart Disease</u>

Another major benefit that makes people take a look at the Ketogenic Diet is the downstream effects of the diet on blood glucose levels. As you begin to cut carbohydrates from your diet, it can help keep your blood glucose stable and low. By doing this, individuals have been able to keep their blood pressure in check and are also able to lower their triglyceride levels.

When people first begin a Ketogenic Diet, they feel that it is counterintuitive to eat a higher percentage of fat in order to lower the triglycerides, but the truth is, fat has had a bad rep this whole time! In fact, it is eating excessive carbohydrates, especially fructose, that is the culprit behind increasing triglycerides! The truth is, through this new diet, you will be able to raise your good cholesterol and lower your bad cholesterol.

<u>Fight Cancer</u>

When it comes to cancer, it is essential that you seek medical attention before you try to take your life into your own hands through diet. It is highly advised that you listen to your doctor's advice when it comes down to cancer treatment. However, there have been articles published based around cancer and the ketogenic diet.

In 2014, Dom D'Agostino's lab published an article based around ketones being able to decrease tumor cell viability in mice that had metastatic cancer. Within this article, it was found that, generally, cancer cells will express an abnormal metabolism that is characterized when glucose consumption is increased. When this happens, the genes begin to mutate, and the mitochondrial begins to malfunction. In the studies, it is found that cancer cells are unable to use ketone bodies as energy, therefore inhibiting the viability of the tumor cell in the first place!

Improve Sleep and Energy Levels

Unfortunately, many individuals underestimate how important sleep is. The good news is that after only four or five days on the ketogenic diet, many individuals have reported that they already begin to benefit from higher energy levels. On a scientific level, this may be due to the fact that through your new ketogenic diet, you will be stabilizing your insulin levels. As your body becomes stabilized, this will help provide you with a ready source of energy rather than experiencing the spikes and crashes.

As far as sleeping goes, the ketogenic diet affects sleep are still being studied. Right now, it seems as though through diet, individuals are able to decrease the time they spend in REM and increase slow-wave sleep patterns. It is believed that this is due to a biochemical shift in the brain as your body learned to use ketones as energy. Either way, you will be sleeping more in-depth and longer than before, granting you a fresh start to each day!

Decrease Inflammation

Inflammation is a strange defense mechanism used in the body to help the immune system recognize any damaged cells, pathogens, or irritants. Through inflammation, the body is able to identify these issues and begin the healing process. While this is beneficial for the most part, it, unfortunately, can persist longer than needed and will end up causing more harm than good.

If you have inflammation in your body, you may experience symptoms such as pain, redness, swelling, immobility, and sometimes even heat. But, these signs of inflammations only apply to the inflammations on the skin. Sometimes, inflammation can happen within our internal organs, and that is when we experience symptoms such as fever, abdominal pain, chest pain, mouth sores, and even fatigue.

Studies have found that the key player in inflammation, and the diseases associated with it, is suppressed BHB. Luckily through the ketogenic diet, BHB is one of the primary ketones you will be producing as you begin your new diet. This meaning that you will be able to help issues, including IBS, eczema, psoriasis, acne, and even arthritis, all through diet!

Gastrointestinal and Gallbladder Health

If you suffer from heartburn or acid reflux on a daily basis, you may want to take a good, hard look at your diet. Unfortunately, many sugary foods, nightshade vegetables, and grain-based foods are major culprits of both heartburn and acid reflux. With that in mind, it shouldn't come as a surprise that when you change your diet to include low-carb foods, these symptoms will disappear almost instantly. The reason you experience these issues is through an autoimmune response, bacterial issue, and inflammation caused by these foods in the first place.

Another benefit of the Ketogenic Diet will be the altering of the microbiome found in your gut. An individual known as Dr. Eric Westman found that through diet, individuals are able to significantly reduce health issues as they change their microbiome. In fact, he believes that when you take away carbohydrates, this can fix just about any gastrointestinal issues that affect a number of different people.

Along those same lines, research has also found that carbohydrates may be a significant culprit behind gallstones as well. As far as the Ketogenic Diet goes, it appears that when individuals consume a diet that is higher in fat, this can help keep the system running smoothly and will prevent gallstones from forming in the first place.

Improved Kidney Function

Another common issue among the health community is kidney stones. The most common cause of both gout and kidney stones is due to elevated levels of phosphorus, oxalate, calcium, and uric acid in the body. Unfortunately, this is often combined with obesity, dehydration, bad genetics, sugar consumption, and alcohol consumption.

Through the Ketogenic diet, individuals are able to lower their uric acid levels and help improve the health of their kidneys. It should be noted that while the ketogenic diet can help long-term, this diet does temporarily raise the uric acid levels within the body, especially if you are dehydrated. While it does rise as the ketone levels rise, the uric acid levels will lower in about four to six weeks.

Improved Women's Health

While the ketogenic diet is beneficial for both men and women, studies have shown that through diet, women may be able to stabilize their hormones and increase their fertility.

There was extensive research published in 2013 that looked at the key evidence linking ketogenic diets to enhancing fertility. It was also found that the Ketogenic Diet can treat PCOS (Polycystic Ovary Syndrome.) Through diet, individuals were able to eliminate or reduce symptoms of PCOS, including obesity, acne, and prolonged menstrual periods.

On a more general basis, it seems as though with this diet, individuals were able to keep their blood sugar levels low and stable. When this happens, it helps stabilize and equilibrate hormone levels, especially in women. Fortunately, this is a downstream benefit of the metabolic pathways that are related to insulin. Overall, individuals feel more balanced and stable than ever!

Improved Endurance and Muscle Gain

As we get older, we generally begin to lose the muscle mass we once had. As mentioned earlier, one of the main ketones you will begin producing as you begin the Ketogenic Diet is BHB. BHB is helpful in promoting muscle gain. When you combine the ketogenic diet with proper exercise, you will be increasing your health and muscle gain at the same time.

In addition to muscle gain, it is also believed that the diet can help improve endurance. Studies have found that athletes who switched to the diet and became fully fat-adapted showed significant improvements in both their mental and physical performances. Of course, this was compared to individuals who followed a typical diet that is rich in carbohydrates.

<u>Weight Loss</u>

Weight loss is one of the major reasons anyone begins a diet. Luckily through the ketogenic diet, there is substantial evidence that by eating the proper foods, you will be able to lose weight and preserve your muscle mass. In a related study, it was found that individuals who followed a ketogenic diet, compared to individuals on a low-calorie and low-fat diet were able to lose 2.2 times more weight! In addition, these people also improved their HDL cholesterol and Triglyceride levels.

The best part about losing weight on the Ketogenic diet is the fact that individuals are still able to lose fat without restricting their calories nor controlling their food intake. This is important to keep in mind when it comes down to sticking to any diet. When individuals hate the extra work of counting their calories, they are statistically more likely to return to their old eating habits. Later in this book, we will be going over the specifics of weight loss on the Ketogenic Diet.

<u>Increased Metabolic Health</u>

The last health benefit we will focus on in this chapter will be increased metabolic health. Metabolic syndrome is described as give common risk factors for heart disease, type 2 diabetes, and obesity. These include high blood sugar levels, low levels of HDL "good" cholesterol, high levels of LDL "bad" cholesterol, abdominal obesity, and high blood pressure. The good news is that many of these risk factors can be eliminated or improved through better lifestyle and nutritional changes.

An important factor behind these issues is insulin. Insulin plays a vital role as far as metabolic disease and diabetes go. Luckily, the Ketogenic Diet is very effective when it comes to lowering insulin levels for individuals who are prediabetic or have type 2 diabetes.

In one study, it was found that after only two weeks following the Ketogenic Diet, individuals were able to improve their insulin sensitivity by 75% and showed a blood sugar level drop from 7.5 mmol/l to a 6.2mmol/l! In another 16-week study, seven out of the 21 participants were able to stop their diabetic medication completely when they began the Ketogenic Diet.

As you can tell, the Ketogenic Diet can help a number of different people. While that is important to know, it is more important to understand how it works. The key to your success is going to be fat! While that may seem backward, what we are taught about fat is all backward! Yes, there are bad fats that we have to avoid, but good fat is going to be your new fuel source. Therefore, we will next learn the different types of fat you need to boost your success on the Ketogenic Diet.

Chapter 3:

How To Start A Keto Diet When You're Over 50?

So once you have made your decision, the next thing to do is speak to your doctor about it. As discussed, whether or not you're suffering from a medical condition, it's important to speak to your doctor to learn more about the keto diet and if it's right for you. Let's take a look at some steps to take when getting started:

1. Do your research on keto-friendly food

First of all, you need to acquire a list of foods to eat and avoid. Depending on your budget and location, some of those foods may be difficult to find. So you may want to look for food alternatives that are also keto-friendly. Also, learn how to spot "hidden carbs" in food items you purchase. Many foods may claim to be keto-friendly but may contain additional carbs or sugars.

2. Practice portion control

Just because you're allowed to eat foods rich in fats and proteins, doesn't mean you should eat excessive amounts. Although you don't have to count calories every time you eat, you should practice portion control, so you don't go overboard. This is where a high-quality food scale comes in handy.

3. Be prepared to experience some side effects

Although these side effects don't happen to most people, you might be one of those unlucky enough to experience them. One of the most common side effects is a condition known as the "keto flu". You will know that you have this condition if you experience side effects such as headaches, fatigue, irritability, a lack of motivation, brain fog (an inability to focus), sugar cravings, muscle cramps, dizziness, and nausea. However, if you already know what to watch out for, then you don't have to worry. Most of these side effects are temporary and will go away. Also, try not to let the side effects discourage you from sticking with the diet.

Tips for Sticking with the Keto Diet

Remember, the keto diet is more than an eating plan; it's a whole new lifestyle. If you want to stick with this diet for the long-term, here are some pointers to keep in mind:

1. Consider your motivation for starting the keto diet

If you want to make this diet plan part of your life, you need to make sure you're doing it for the right reasons. If you're just starting the diet to join the trend, chances are, you might give up at the first sign of difficulty. However, if you have a good reason to follow the diet and you're sure that it will motivate you, then there's a good chance you will follow through. Some of the common reasons why people start this diet include the following:

Incorporating the diet as part of the treatment plan for certain conditions. For instance, inflammation, diabetes, heart disease, brain-related disorders, and even cancer.

To lose weight, especially for those who have a hard time losing fat.

To achieve and stay in a state of ketosis.

2. Learn how to count your macros

This is especially important at the start of your journey. As time goes by, you will learn how to estimate your meals without having to use a food scale.

3. Prepare your kitchen for your keto-friendly foods

Once you've made the choice, it's time to get rid of all the foods in your kitchen that aren't allowed in the keto diet. To do this, check the nutritional labels of all the food items. Of course, there's no need to throw everything away. You can donate foods you don't need to food kitchens and other institutions that give food to the needy.

4. Purchase some keto strips for yourself

These are important so you can check your ketone levels and track of your progress. You can purchase keto strips in pharmacies and online. For instance, some of the best keto strips available on Amazon are Perfect Keto Ketone Test Strips, Smackfat Ketone Strips, and One Earth Ketone Strips.

These are important for beginners, but if you have already been following the diet for some time, you will learn how to determine when your body is in ketosis just by how you're feeling.

5. Download a keto diet app to help you with your journey

These days, there are apps for everything! If you need to find more motivation to keep you on the path to a keto lifestyle, you can download an app for yourself. There are plenty of apps available, and they all have their own features. Research about these apps to find out which app would be the best one for you.

Here are a few great keto apps you can try:

MyFitnessPal: This app has more than 150 million registered users now. It's one of the most popular apps out there, and it also has its own website. With this app, you can keep track of your macros and determine your best nutrient and calorie intake based on your own personal health goals.

Keto Diet: You can think of this app as your own personal keto sidekick. Use it to keep track of your weight as well as your macros. With it, you can find out how the changes you're making in your diet are affecting your body.

Carb Manager: This is another excellent keto companion as it has a database of over a million foods along with their macronutrient, micronutrient, and net carbohydrate information. Using this app makes it easier for you to shop for the foods to incorporate into your daily meals.

6. Ask your doctor if you need to take supplements

Whether you're completely healthy or have an existing medical condition, it's important to speak with your doctor first before you start. That way, you can learn more about the diet, ask any questions, and look for recommendations for supplements you can take to complement your keto diet.

7. Have the proper mindset

Your mindset is one of the most important things you need to change when you've decided to follow the keto lifestyle. Without the right mindset, you might not stick with the diet long enough to enjoy all its benefits. Also, the proper mindset will keep you motivated to keep going no matter what challenges come your way. Here are some tips to help you achieve the proper mindset to achieve success:

Think of your motivation or the reasons why you want to start the keto diet. If you think it will help, list out these reasons and refer back to them when you're feeling challenged.

Make a list of your health goals - both the simple ones that are easily achievable and the significant ones that require more time and effort.

Do a lot of research to learn about the keto diet so you know exactly how you will approach this new lifestyle.

Chapter 4:

How Does Aging Affect Your Nutritional Needs

Nutrition is vital to maintain health and to lead an active and fulfilling life. There is another fact that your nutritional need changes throughout your life and that's why eating healthy becomes more important. If you are eating unhealthy food and suffering from nutritional deficiencies, then this will bring harmful outcomes, and you will lead a poor-quality life.

Childhood: In the initial years of life, the little bodies need essential nutrients along with regular nutrients to ensure they develop and grow physically and mentally. The food should provide high energy to support the rapid growth of bodies at this age. Also, childhood is the time of learning and experiencing new foods and developing taste and smell sense, which shape their eating habits for later in life. Therefore, children should be encouraged to consume a variety of foods every day. The key nutrient in children's diet includes protein which is necessary for growth, calcium and vitamin D to grow strong bones. Adolescence: The body around this time goes through significant emotional and physical changes due to puberty. Moreover, maturing sexuality increases the muscles growth and strengthens the bones, and this is a perfect opportunity for children to build strong bones for later. For this reason, it is really essential that the body meets its calcium requirement. For this, dairy milk products are perfect healthy choices such as yogurt, milk, and cheese that are well known for high-quality protein and calcium-rich sources. Iron is an also essential bone nutrient that can be obtained from red meat, chicken, kidney beans, spinach, and mussels.

Encourage them to have water or milk as beverages and healthy snacks to combat craving and untimely hunger. Also, make-ahead some smoothies, prepare grab-and-go food options like toasts and sandwiches and do meal prepping for children that can't sit long enough to eat food at the meal table.

Adulthood: This is the time when you have to focus on maintaining the healthy body you have developed through your childhood and adolescence. Therefore, the body should get good enough nutrition like protein, calcium, vitamins, and phosphorus that helps you stay active, energetic and maintain bones and muscles that tend to decrease as we move forward in age. Focus on eating healthy foods that give you all the nutrients, which make you feel great without disturbing your ideal body weight and reduce the factors of ailments like diabetes and heart diseases.

Older age: At the old age, the body needs same or even more protein, minerals, and vitamins. For example, after the age of 50, your body's ability to absorb specific vitamins fades due to hormonal changes, and you don't have enough stomach acid to break down food sources. So, if you aren't eating foods that don't have these vitamins or not taking nutrients supplements then you may suffer from dangerous ailments. Also, you may eat less than previously due to reduced appetite, health issues or medications. In that case, eat little and often can effectively help your body in getting essential nutrients that support mobility, active mind, growth, mental and physical performance. Enjoy a variety of foods and drinks and go for nutritious and natural options for foods that contain a range of nutrients. Similarly, you may not notice thirst in your later years, but keeping your body hydrated is important at any age. With these examples, you have to make little bits of changes in what you eat and drink to achieve optimal health no matter what your age is.

There are many scientific theories out there that explain how the human body ages and deteriorates over time, two of which are free radical theory of aging and glycation theory of aging.

The free radical theory explains that our body becomes damaged because of the free radicals trying to bind to the molecules in our body in their search for more electron, which leads to damage and inflammation. In the process of binding, your molecule becomes unstable and binds with your other molecule to get its electron, and the cycle repeats in a process known as oxidation, causing a lot of damage over time. The solution this theory proposed is to increase your body's pool of antioxidants because they have an extra electron to give to the free radicals in your body, thus preventing them from taking and destabilizing your body's molecules.

The glycation theory of aging proposes that we age because of the glycation damage from high blood sugar. That means the excess sugar in the body clings onto the proteins in the body, preventing them from doing their jobs, which can lead to many complications, one of which is diabetes.

But how does the keto diet come in? Keto diets can help the body slow the aging process in many ways:

1.   Keto diet minimizes damages done by oxidation and increases the body's store of uric acid and other antioxidants.

2.   Ketosis increases the mitochondrial glutathione, which is a potent antioxidant that resides within the mitochondria, the powerhouse of your cell. Antioxidants that are digested orally are not very effective in protecting your cells. But ketosis supports the cell directly.

3.   Keto diets are very low in sugar, meaning that your blood sugar level would be much lower, reducing the chance of glycation damages.

4.   Keto diets are low in carbs, which improves blood sugar control level and suppress appetite because they have the same effects as fasting.

5.   Keto diets also reduce triglycerides, which are the fatty acids in the bloodstream that are used to measure heart disease risk. You want triglycerides in your body to be as low as possible.

In short, keto diets reduce your blood sugar level, prevent glycation damages, and inflammation. These three conditions are associated with all sorts of diseases that lead to death. Therefore, keto diets ate the best way to reduce blood sugar and insulin levels, increase your longevity and wellbeing.

Chapter 5:

Benefits of The Keto Diet For People Over 50

So what exactly can you look forward to once you go on a Ketogenic Diet? There are tons of benefits! Here are some of the pros of this brand-new diet:

<u>Efficient Way to Lose Weight</u>

Let's forget calories for a few minutes and just concentrate on the kind of nutrients you have in your food. A study published in PubMed which allows for a meta-analysis of randomized controlled trial between a very-low carbohydrate ketogenic diet versus a low-fat diet for long term weight loss shows that the low-carb option provides for better long-term results. It can even help reduce risk factors of cardiovascular problems, which simply means that you'll have less chances of suffering from heart problems or high blood pressure. The science behind this isn't that complicated. The fact is that the body finds it easier to turn sugar into energy – which is why when given the choice, your body will always choose to run on sugar. Fat is also a possible source of energy – but it takes more work, which is why you lose weight more consistently with a Ketogenic Diet.

<u>Reduces the Risk of Acne</u>

You'd think a person in their 50's wouldn't have acne – and you'd probably be right. Note though that a large part of what you eat affects skin health, even if you're already in your 50s. In fact, people in their 50s need to be extra careful with skin health because this is when growths, blackheads, pore blockages, and more become persistent. Studies show that rapid changes in blood sugar have an effect on skin health as discussed in a study titled: Nutrition and acne – therapeutic potential of ketogenic diets.

May Help Reduce Cancer Risks

Switching to the Ketogenic Diet may help reduce the risk of cancer, especially as the risk of it increases upon reaching the age of 50. Although that's just a small percentage, it's definitely worth noting – especially if you happen to have a history of cancer in the family. It's also interesting to note that the Ketogenic Diet is usually prescribed as a complement to chemotherapy. A study titled "Ketogenic diets as an adjuvant cancer therapy: history and potential mechanism" concluded that the deprivation of sugar causes more stress to the cancer cells. This simply means that cancer cells depend more on the glucose you have on your body and once their energy source is cut-off, they're more likely to die off.

Reduces Risk of Heart Problems

Healthy fat found in avocado, nuts, and other food items promoted by the Ketogenic Diet can help reduce the possibility of heart problems. In a study titled: The long-term effects of a ketogenic diet in obese patients, it was seen that going on a Keto Diet significantly increases HDL and lowers LDL. HDL is known as the "good cholesterol" while LDL is the "bad cholesterol" known for increasing the likelihood of heart problems. The bad type are still discouraged and are not part of the Ketogenic Diet.

Protects Brain Function

Have you ever found yourself trying to remember simple things – like what things to buy from the store or what day to pay the power bill? Forgetfulness becomes more common as you grow older – but it doesn't have to be! In a study titled: The effects of Ketogenic Diet on behavior and cognition, it was revealed that children following the diet have better cognitive functioning and alertness. It's also theorized that the diet has neurological protective benefits – which basically means that it can help prevent problems that affect brain function. For example, you'll have slightly lower risks of Parkinson's, Alzheimer's, and other forms of dementia.

Bone Health

Osteoporosis becomes more likely as a person advances in age. This is especially true if you weren't able to introduce appropriate amounts of calcium in your body. As you probably known, osteoporosis makes the bone brittle and fragile. This means that your likelihood of having serious injury from seemingly small accidents increases. A simple slip and bones can fracture or hips may become dislocated. Persistent inflammation of the joints could become an everyday problem. The Ketogenic Diet is a good way of preventing these from happening because the diet naturally involves the intake of healthy dairy or milk products. More importantly, the Ketogenic Diet promotes the intake of low-toxin food products. Hence, your body absorbs food nutrients better, ensuring that all the minerals you need is distributed evenly throughout the body.

But I'm Over 50!

I understand that you have several concerns when using the Ketogenic Diet. Sure, the benefits are definitely great – but many of these benefits are experienced by those who are in their 40s or younger. This means that aside from the excess weight, they don't really have any other health problems to contend with. But what if you're already in your 50s or more? From what I see, most people in their 50s already have several health issues. Usually, these are health problems that occur simply because of age – so don't feel too bad about yourself!

For example, high blood pressure, heart problems, and diabetes are common problems for people in their 50s. If you happen to be this situation – it's important to first consult your doctor before going on the Ketogenic Diet – or any other diet for that matter. Since we're doing our best to cover all areas of Ketogenic Diet for people over 50, this book will also talk about some of the downsides if you have existing health problems. As someone who has done extensive research and have a ton of personal experiences from working with clients, I want you to know that there is absolutely NOTHING to be afraid of when switching to this brand new dietary plan.

Chapter 6:

Keto Side Effects and How to Salve Them

It would be very irresponsible of me if I only tell you all the good things about the Ketogenic Diet and ignore the side effects. The truth is that there are negative effects that could happen once you start the Ketogenic Diet – but that's actually true for all of them! All types of diet have negative effects to start with because your body has gotten used to the bad habits. Once you make the shift to a more positive way of eating, the body sort of goes on a rebellious phase so it feels like everything is going wrong. For example, a person who used to eat lots of sugar in a day can have severe headaches once they start to avoid the sugar. This is a withdrawal symptom and tells you that your diet is actually making positive changes to the body – albeit it takes a little bit of pain on your part.

So what can one expect when they make that change towards a healthy Ketogenic Diet? Here are some of the things to expect and of course – how to troubleshoot these problems.

Long Term Side Effects

A study titled "Metabolic Effects of the Very Low Carbohydrate Diets: Misunderstood Villains of Human Metabolism" shows that for short-term purposes, the Ketogenic Diet is very effective. It lets you burn all those excess fat quickly but in a healthy way. If you do this for a long period of time however, there will be side effects. For example, there can be muscle loss, dizziness, kidney problems, acidosis, and problems with focus. Does that mean you shouldn't go on a Ketogenic Diet at all? Of course not! This only means that you'll have to be careful when using this diet. Don't push it too hard and you will be able to get all the positive results with none of the downsides!

Do you know why a low carbohydrate diet is bad if done for a long time? Well, balance is important in anything you do and the Ketogenic Diet doesn't really support balance. If you get rid of an entire food group for a long period of time, your body will rebel against you. Remember – the Ketogenic Diet relies on stored fat in your body. If there are no more stored fat, it really won't work anymore so you will have to increase your carbohydrates. To solve this problem, I recommend going on a 30-day Ketogenic Diet first and assessing your health before moving forward. Asking your doctor what to do "next" after the 30-day plan or after hitting your weight goal is also a good idea. Personally, I decided to increase my carbohydrate intake slightly after hitting my goal weight.

<u>Keto Flu</u>

The Keto Flu is the most prominent problem you'll encounter when starting the diet. It's a perfectly normal reaction by the body that may seem alarming because, well, the symptoms don't really feel good. You have to understand, your body has been running on a specific type of gasoline for years. It's been taking fuel from sugar and with the Ketogenic Diet, it's like you're changing your fuel source to a cleaner and more sustainable type. It makes sense that the engine growls a little in protest – but after that, you'll be able to run beautifully without the guilt.

The Keto Flu has the following symptoms:

Headaches

Fatigue

Irritability

Brain fog or difficulty focusing

Motivational problems

Sugar cravings

Dizziness

Nausea

Muscle cramps

Frequent urination

These symptoms are all heavily dependent on the kind of person doing the Keto Diet. Since you're already in our 50s, the symptoms may be more prominent, especially if you rely heavily on carbohydrates in your diet. If you eat mostly low-carb food however, these effects may not be as obvious.

But how do you solve them? Here are some of the best way to get rid of the Keto Flu as quickly as possible!

First, increase your water and salt consumption. This happens a lot once you start a Ketogenic Diet. You may not notice it, but a lot of the salt you consume is through carbohydrates like bread, pasta, rice, and so on. Salt tends to make you thirsty so if you eat little salt, you're also less likely to look for water during the day. So what happens now? Every time you feel dizzy or tired or nauseous while on a Keto Diet, just dissolve salt in water and gulp it down. Now, this is not going to taste good - but I promise that it will help you feel better. You can always try consuming the salt and water separately – whatever you find most convenient. As for water, try to hit a target of 3 liters of water every day. The good news is that this doesn't have to be plain water – your smoothies, coffee, and tea drinks are also counted.

Add more fat in your diet. Because of all the wrong information circulating today, a lot of people are afraid of fat. We've discussed this before but it bears repeating – fat is not your enemy. During the Ketogenic Diet, it makes sense to eat lots of fats especially if your carbohydrate intake dips to an all-time low. If you lower the carbohydrate consumption without an equal fat increase, then you will always feel hungry and tired.

Don't be impatient – go slower. Remember what we said about the body changing fuels when you're switching to the Ketogenic Diet? Well, the changing process doesn't have to be overnight. Choose to convert one meal at a time to a Keto-friendly set instead of changing all of them on your first day. Of course, it's recommended that you only do this if the salt water method doesn't for you. Just remember – the Keto Flu will pass so the first few days of discomfort should not discourage you in the slightest. If you want to minimize the trouble, try starting your Ketogenic Diet on a low-stress period – like a holiday. So basically, instead of eating less than 50 grams of carbohydrates a day, you can have a target of 50 to 70.

Do NOT count calories or restrict your food consumption. When it comes to the Ketogenic Diet – you don't have to calorie count. Again, you don't want to just stuff yourself with food just because you don't have to count calories, but the truth is calories do not matter so much when your body is at a state of Ketosis. It doesn't matter so much how many you're getting – your body will always break down the fat deposits and there will be weight loss. Stressing about the calorie intake or depriving yourself of food because of the calories can actually worsen the symptoms of Keto Flu and will make it more difficult for you to stick to the diet. The bottom line is this: as long as you're eating the allowed food items in allowed portions, then you're OK.

Limit your physical activity. That's the good news with the Ketogenic Diet – you don't have to exercise. Sure, you may not be running marathons or going to the gym on a weekly basis, but if you're health-conscious, then chances are you do light walks on a routine basis. That's perfectly OK – as long as you don't over-exert yourself. Now, there will be days when you will actually feel too good. Like you can go out and exercise because you have all this extra energy. When this happens, resist the temptation to do too much too soon. Your body is already burning as much fat as it can – don't push it too hard or you might get sick. If you're restless, try doing yoga, light walking, or just stretching.

Take some supplements. People using the Ketogenic Diet for a long time may also have vitamin and mineral deficiency. It's not easily obvious but it could happen so you'll have to be prepared. The usual vitamins and minerals lacking in a Ketogenic Diet include calcium, zinc, selenium, and vitamin D – so try taking a multivitamin during your diet. Again, I can't stress this enough: always consult your doctor before taking any sort of medication. This is especially true if you have pre-existing health problems and are also taking medication for maintenance.

<u>Constipation or Diarrhea</u>

These problems are fairly common because, well, you're changing your diet! Your body will react one way or another and in both cases, the solution is practically the same – water and fiber. Make sure you get enough fluids in your system and take fiber supplements which is available through many stores. You can also try taking laxatives that are made especially without carbohydrates.

If alarming symptoms occurs while you're on the Ketogenic Diet, I want you to consult your doctor ASAP! Again, reactions may vary from one person to the next and I don't want you shrugging off certain symptoms as if they're just "part" of the diet. Stay motivated but also be mindful of what is happening to your body. Remember – we want you to be healthy!

Chapter 7:

Keto Grocery List

I've had people complain about the difficulty of switching their grocery list to one that's Ketogenic-friendly. The fact is that food is expensive – and most of the food you have in your fridge are probably packed full with carbohydrates. This is why if you're committing to a Ketogenic Diet, you need to do a clean sweep. That's right – everything that's packed with carbohydrates should be identified and set aside to make sure you're not eating more than you should. You can donate them to a charity before going out and buying your new Keto-friendly shopping list.

<u>Seafood</u>

Seafood means fish like sardines, mackerel, and wild salmon. It's also a good idea to add some shrimp, tuna, mussels, and crab into your diet. This is going to be a tad expensive but definitely worth it in the long run. What's the common denominator in all these food items? The secret is omega-3 fatty acids which is credited for lots of health benefits. You want to add food rich in omega-3 fatty acids in your diet.

<u>Low-carb Vegetables</u>

Not all vegetables are good for you when it comes to the Ketogenic Diet. The vegetable choices should be limited to those with low carbohydrate counts. Pack up your cart with items like spinach, eggplant, arugula, broccoli, and cauliflower. You can also put in bell peppers, cabbage, celery, kale, Brussels sprouts, mushrooms, zucchini, and fennel.

So what's in them? Well, aside from the fact that they're low-carb, these vegetable also contain loads of fiber which makes digestion easier. Of course, there's also the presence of vitamins, minerals, antioxidants, and various other nutrients that you need for day to day life. Which ones should you avoid? Steer clear of the starch-packed vegetables like carrots, turnips, and beets. As a rule, you go for the vegetables that are green and leafy.

Fruits Low in Sugar

During an episode of sugar-craving, it's usually a good idea to pick low-sugar fruit items. Believe it or not, there are lots of those in the market! Just make sure to stock up on any of these: avocado, blackberries, raspberries, strawberries, blueberries, lime, lemon, and coconut. Also note that tomatoes are fruits too so feel free to make side dishes or dips with loads of tomatoes! Keep in mind that these fruits should be eaten fresh and not out of a can. If you do eat them fresh off the can however, take a good look at the nutritional information at the back of the packaging. Avocadoes are particularly popular for those practicing the Ketogenic Diet because they contains LOTS of the good kind of fat.

Meat and Eggs

While some diets will tell you to skip the meat, the Ketogenic Diet actually encourages its consumption. Meat is packed with protein that will feed your muscles and give you a consistent source of energy through the day. It's a slow but sure burn when you eat protein as opposed to carbohydrates which are burned faster and therefore stored faster if you don't use them immediately.

But what kind of meat should you be eating? There's chicken, beef, pork, venison, turkey, and lamb. Keep in mind that quality plays a huge role here – you should be eating grass-fed organic beef or organic poultry if you want to make the most out of this food variety. The organic option lets you limit the possibility of ingesting toxins in your body due to the production process of these products. Plus, the preservation process also means there are added salt or sugar in the meat, which can throw off the whole diet.

Nuts and Seeds

Nuts and seeds you should definitely add in your cart include: chia seeds, brazil nuts, macadamia nuts, flaxseed, walnuts, hemp seeds, pecans, sesame seeds, almonds, hazelnut, and pumpkin seeds. They also contain lots of protein and very little sugar so they're great if you have the munchies. They're the ideal snack because they're quick, easy, and will keep you full. They're high in calories though, which is why lots of people steer clear of them. As I mentioned earlier though – the Ketogenic Diet has nothing to do with calories and everything to do with the nutrient you're eating. So don't pay too much attention on the calorie count and just remember that they're a good source of fats and protein.

Dairy Products

OK – some people in their 50s already have a hard time processing dairy products, but for those who don't – you can happily add many of these to your diet. Make sure to consume sufficient amounts of cheese, plain Greek yogurt, cream butter, and cottage cheese. These dairy products are packed with calcium, protein, and the healthy kind of fat.

Oils

Nope, we're not talking about essentials oils but rather, MCT oil, coconut oil, avocado oil, nut oils, and even extra-virgin olive oil. You can start using those for your frying needs to create healthier food options. The beauty of these oils is that they add flavor to the food, making sure you don't get bored quickly with the recipes. Try picking up different types of Keto-friendly oils to add some variety to your cooking.

Coffee and Tea

The good news is that you don't have to skip coffee if you're going on a Ketogenic Diet. The bad news is that you can't go to Starbucks anymore and order their blended coffee choices. Instead, beverages would be limited to unsweetened tea or unsweetened coffee in order to keep the sugar consumption low. Opt for organic coffee and tea products to make the most out of these powerful antioxidants.

Dark Chocolate

Yes – chocolate is still on the menu, but it is limited to just dark chocolate. Technically, this means eating chocolate that is 70 percent cacao, which would make the taste a bit bitter.

Sugar Substitutes

Later in the recipes part of this book, you might be surprised at some of the ingredients required in the list. This is because while sweeteners are an important part of food preparation, you can't just use any kind of sugar in your recipe. Remember: the typical sugar is pure carbohydrate. Even if you're not eating carbohydrates, if you're dumping lots of sugar in your food – you're not really following the Ketogenic Diet principles.

So what do you do? You find sugar substitutes. The good news is that there are LOTS of those in the market. You can get rid of the old sugar and use any of these as a good substitute.

Stevia. This is perhaps the most familiar one in this list. It's a natural sweetener derived from plants and contains very few calories. Unlike your typical sugar, stevia may actually help lower the sugar levels instead of causing it to spike. Note though that it's sweeter than actual sugar so when cooking with stevia, you'll need to lower the amount used. Typically, the ratio is 200 grams of sugar per 1 teaspoon of powdered stevia.

Sucralose. It contains zero calories and zero carbohydrates. It's actually an artificial sweetener and does not metabolize – hence the complete lack of carbohydrates. Splenda is actually a sweetener derived from sucralose. Note though that you don't want to use this as a baking substitute for sugar. Its best use is for coffee, yogurt, and oatmeal sweetening. Note though that like stevia, it's also very sweet – in fact, it's actually 600 times sweeter than the typical sugar. Use sparingly.

Erythritol. It's a naturally occurring compound that interacts with the tongue's sweet taste receptors. Hence, it mimics the taste of sugar without actually being sugar. It does contain calories, but only about 5% of the calories you'll find in the typical sugar. Note though that it doesn't dissolve very well so anything prepared with this sweetener will have a gritty feeling. This can be problematic if you're using the product for baking. As for sweetness, the typical ratio is 1 1/3 cup for 1 cup of sugar.

Xylitol. Like erythritol, xylitol is a type of sugar alcohol that's commonly used in sugar-free gum. While it still contains calories, the calories are just 3 per gram. It's a sweetener that's good for diabetic patients because it doesn't raise the sugar levels or insulin in the body. The great thing about this is that you don't have to do any computations when using it for baking, cooking, or fixing a drink. The ratio of it with sugar is 1 to 1 so you can quickly make the substitution in the recipe.

What About Condiments?

Condiments are still on the table, but they won't be as tasty as you're used to. Your options include mustard, olive oil mayonnaise, oil-based salad dressings, and unsweetened ketchup. Of all these condiments, ketchup is the one with the most sugar, so make a point of looking for one with reduced sugar content. Or maybe avoid ketchup altogether and stick to mustard?

What About Snacks?

The good news is that there are packed snacks for those who don't have the time to make it themselves. Sugarless nut butters, dried seaweeds, nuts, and sugar-free jerky are all available in stores. The nuts and seeds discussed in a previous paragraph all make for excellent snack options.

What About Labels?

Let's not fool ourselves into thinking that we can cook food every single day. The fact is that there will be days when there will be purchases for the sake of convenience. There are also instances when you'll have problems finding the right ingredients for a given recipe. Hence, you'll need to find substitutes for certain ingredients without losing the "Keto friendly" vibe of the product.

So what should be done? Well, you need to learn how to read labels. Food doesn't have to be specially made to be keto-friendly, you just have to make sure that it doesn't contain any of the unfriendly nutrients or that the carbohydrate content is low enough.

Here's a step by step procedure on how to make a decision based on the labels:

1.   First, take a good look at the ingredient list. You can usually find this at the bottom portion of the label and properly designated as "Ingredients".

2.   The first step is to look at the sugar ingredient. If it's listed as one of the first five ingredients, then that already means there's too much sugar in the product to be keto friendly. Note though that sugar comes with many names. The words: glucose, fructose, maltose, lactose, dextrose, corn syrup and more, are all indicative of sugar content. You'd want to make sure they're not listed within the first 5 ingredients of the food product you're buying. That's one of the best things about the food industry – they're required to list ingredients in the order of quantity so that the first ones listed have more volume in the product.

3.   If the food passes the "sugar" test, you should next look at the carbohydrate content.

4.   You'll notice that carbohydrates are often broken down into groups. Hence, labels may indicate that total carbohydrates are 5grams and then right below that, you can see Dietary Fiber at 1gram and Sugar at 1gram. The important thing to note here is that the dietary fiber and the sugar are part of the total carbohydrates.

5.   Why is this important? Well, most people count the total carbohydrates when computing their carbohydrate consumption for the day. Hence, if your goal is to eat less than 50grams of carbohydrates during the day, then you'll be computing using the 5gram amount.

6.   Some people however make use of the "net carbohydrates" when computing their consumption. Net carbohydrates are what you get when you subtract the other carbohydrate sources from the total carbohydrates. Hence, 5 grams less 1 gram for the fiber and another gram for sugar mean that you'll have 3 grams of net carbohydrates.

7.   Again – why is this important? The main distinction occurs for people who have diabetes. It's all about the insulin levels. At the end of the day however, it's all about the 50 grams of carbohydrates limitation in your diet. If you want to stay on the safe side however, then counting the total carbohydrates is usually the best option.

8.   Look at the serving size. Most people think that the Nutrition in the packet refers to all the food items in the pack – but that's not the case at all. The nutritional information is per serving so you'd want to make sure that the carbohydrate content you picture in your head is equal to the food you usually eat in one sitting. For example, a packet of nuts contains 5 serving in total, each serving containing around 5 grams of carbohydrates. If you eat 2 servings in one sitting, then you'll have to remember that you're consuming 10 grams instead of just 5.

Once you've figured this out, you can quickly make calculations in your head about carbohydrate content of what you're eating based on the labels. You will find that this can be easily adjusted to your eating habits so that you always know what you're consuming even if you're not following a set recipe.

Chapter 8:

Let's Talk About Products

Allowed Product List

If you've decided to go on Keto after 50, be sure you won't regret your choice! So when you start something new, the first and the main thing you need to do is consult the Keto dietary features. But most importantly, you must look at the list of allowed products to remember this list and adhere strictly to it.

Don't worry! The low-carb eating plan isn't overly limited. Check out what products you can and must buy in the supermarket and start a new phase in your life.

Meat and Poultry

Chicken, beef, pork, lamb, turkey, veal include no carb, but high protein and fat intake. That is the primary reason why meat and poultry products are known as the staples for the Ketogenic diet. Besides this, bacon and organ meats are also allowed for consumption.

Seafood

When it comes to seafood, you also have an excellent list. You can buy and cook a lot of delicious dishes from:

Lobster

Shrimp

Octopus

Salmon

Tuna

Oysters

Mussels

Squid

Scallops

The most useful Keto seafood is the crab and shrimp. They don't contain carbohydrates at all.

Vegetables

Only low-carb and non-starchy veggies can be eaten by the people who go on the Keto diet. This means that you can add the following vegetables:

Avocados

Tomatoes

Cucumbers

Zucchini

Radishes

Mushrooms

Eggplant

Celery

Bell peppers

Herbs

Asparagus

Kohlrabi

Mustard

Spinach

Lettuce

Kale

Brussel sprouts

Dairy Products

You should be careful with dairy. Not all dairy food can be useful for you if you want to stick to the Keto diet. Here are the products you can buy and cook:

Eggs

Butter and ghee

Heavy cream and whipping cream

Sour cream

Unflavored Greek yogurt

Cottage cheese

Hard, semi-hard, soft, and cream cheeses

Berries

Unfortunately, most fruits have high levels of carbs and can't be included on the Keto diet. However, you can consume:

Blackberries

Raspberries

Strawberries

Blueberries

Nuts and Seeds

A lot of experts recommend paying attention to nuts and seeds that are high-fat and low-carb. You can add such nuts and seeds to your dishes as:

Almond

Pecans

Walnuts

Hazelnuts

Brazil nuts

Pumpkin seeds

Sesame seeds

Chia seeds

Flaxseed

Coconut and Olive Oils

To cook tasty fatty dishes, you need oil. Coconut and olive oils have unique properties that make them suitable for a Keto diet. These oils are rich in fat and boost ketone production. Moreover, they can be used for salad dressing and adding to cooked dishes.

Low-Carb Drinks

The Keto diet means that you should drink only unsweetened coffee and tea because they don't include carbs and fasten metabolism. Besides, you can drink dark chocolate and cocoa. Such drinks have low levels of carbohydrates and that's why they're permitted.

Prohibited Product List

When it comes to the lists of foods you should avoid on the low-carb, high-fat diet, be attentive and check it carefully. Well, you can't eat:

Grains (like oatmeal, pasta, bulgur, corn, wheat, buckwheat, rice, etc.)

Low-fat dairy (fat-free yogurt, skim milk, skim Mozzarella, etc.)

Most fruits (melon, watermelon, apples, peaches, bananas, grapes, oranges, plums, grapefruits, mangos, cherries, pineapples, pears, etc.)

Starchy veggies (potatoes, beets, turnips, parsnips, etc.)

Grain foods (pasta, popcorn, muesli, cereal, bagels, bread, etc.)

Some oils (soyabean oil, grapeseed oil, sunflower oil, peanut oil, canola oil)

Typical snack foods (crackers, potato chips, etc.)

Trans fats (margarine)

Sweets (candies, buns, pastries, cakes, chocolate, puddings, cookies)

Sweeteners and added sugars (corn syrup, cane sugar, honey, agave nectar, etc.)

Sweetened drinks (sweetened coffee and tea, juice, soda, smoothies)

Alcohol (sweet wines, cider, beer, etc.)

Chapter 9:

Exercises to Assist with Quality of Life After 50

The ways that you take care of your body and the ways you stay active will dictate your quality of life and how good you will look. If you do not take care of your body, you might be fifty years old and look like you are sixty-five years old. But if you do good things for your body you might be sixty-five years old and look like you are fifty years old. Age really is just a number. And even if you haven't been active in a long time, or ever, it is never too late to start on some sort of activity plan to increase the quality of your life.

I call it an activity plan because no one really wants to exercise, right? So, let's think of this as an activity plan or a workout routine, both of those are positive statements that say you care about your body and you want to fight the effects of growing older with everything you've got.

Once a woman crosses that fifty-year mark, she begins losing one percent of her muscle each year. But muscle tone and fiber do not need to be lost with aging. With a proper workout, you can continue to build new muscle and maintain what you already have until you are in your nineties. And some of the exercises that you do for your muscles will help you build strong bones. This is especially important for women because losing the estrogen supplies in our bodies will cause us to lose bone mass faster than men do. This is when we are really at risk for developing osteoporosis.

And regular physical activity will help you to avoid developing that middle-age spread around the abdomen or to lose it if you already have it. Activity will help you to maintain a proper weight for your height and build which in turn will help you to avoid many, if not all, of the age-related, obesity-related diseases such as cardiovascular diseases and diabetes.

Physical activity comes in four main types. Each one should be done at least once or twice a week to ensure your body is getting the right mix of activity. The four main types of activity are:

Balance – Older people lose their sense of balance. It is easy for an older person to fall and break something, like a hip. When you engage in activities that help you to maintain your sense of balance will help reduce the risk that you might fall and suffer a permanent injury.

Stretching – As we age our muscles begin to lose their elasticity. This is part of why rolling out of bed in the morning gets more difficult as we get older. Stretching activities will help you to improve and maintain your level of flexibility which will help you to avoid injuries to your joints and muscles.

Cardiovascular/Aerobic – These are also called endurance activities because you should be able to maintain them for at least ten minutes at a time. This key here is to get your heart working faster and your breathing to be deeper. You should be working hard but still able to carry on a conversation. These activities will strengthen your heart and lungs which are, after all, very important muscles in your body.

Strength training – We are not talking about bodybuilding, but if you want to go for it. This will include working out with resistance bands or lifting weights. Either activity will help to build muscle.

While there are four separate categories of exercise that does not mean that you need to keep them strictly separated because many activities will encompass work in more than one area. You can lift light weights while doing balance activities. Walking and swimming will build muscle strength and cardiovascular health. Yoga will improve balance and assist with building muscle strength and stretching. The key is to engage in seventy-five minutes of vigorous activity each week, or fifteen minutes five days each week; or you can get one hundred fifty minutes of moderate activity in five thirty-minute sessions each week.

And make sure that you design a plan that fits you. Remember that it is perfectly fine to change your routine as your needs change. Maybe, in the beginning, you will work on balance three days each week because you really need help with that. But after a few weeks, your balance has improved enough so that you can devote one of those days to strength training. This is your routine made just for you so make it work for you. And don't forget to get your doctor's okay before beginning any type of activity routine. He will most likely give you his blessings but it is always good to ask. He can also provide you with information on activities that are good for you personally.

One thing to note here, especially if you have not been active in a while, is not to begin a vigorous level of activity the same day you begin the keto diet. During the time your body is getting used to the diet and going through ketosis, you will not feel like indulging in a lot of extra activity and your workout routine will be doomed to failure. This journey is all about making you the best you possibly can so don't sabotage yourself in the first few weeks. If you really want to start your activities on day one of your diet then I recommend walking or bicycling. Either of these activities can be started slowly, so a gentle walk or bike around the neighborhood after dinner is a perfect activity.

If you can get out and join a class at a local senior center, YMCA, community college, or church then do that. You will meet new people, some in your age group, and you can all work together to create your new bodies. But taking a class will not be the best choice for everyone. So we have included some basic exercises that can be done in the privacy of your home to get you started on the new lean you.

Stretching – Stretching activities are so important for older adults. These activities will also help you to improve your balance because you might find yourself standing or reaching in new and different ways.

Quad stretch – This is a simple exercise that can be done at home. Hold onto a chair or your partner for balance assistance if you need it. Then with the opposite hand lift the foot on that side behind you. Pull upward gently you can feel the beginning of a stretch in the front of your leg. As people get older, they may lean forward for balance and this muscle, the quad, can become shorter and less efficient over time. Hold this position steady for at least thirty seconds and repeat on the other side.

Hamstring stretch – This activity can be done on the sofa, the bed, or on the floor. Lay one leg in front of you and point your toes to the ceiling. Slowly fold your body over until you feel a stretching in the back of your leg and hold it for thirty seconds. NOTE: if you have recently had a hip replacement check with your doctor before doing this one.

Calf stretch – Place your hands on the wall and step back with one foot. The back foot should be flat on the floor and the front knee should be slightly bent. Then lean forward toward the wall until you feel a stretch in your calf muscle. Hold it for thirty seconds and repeat on the other leg.

BALANCING – Balancing activities are so important for older adults to reduce the risk of falls. Tai Chi and Yoga are both excellent activities for assisting with better balance. You can find DVDs, routines online, or classes taught by certified instructors. Just remember to work with your body and your current level of ability and don't try to do an advanced routine if you have never mastered a beginner routine. You will just be setting yourself up for failure and we are here to succeed. And keep in mind that flexibility activities also help with the effects of arthritis. While you will want to explore the different types of yoga before making a decision on the one that is best for you, here is a yoga pose that anyone can do at home and helps to wake the whole body in the morning.

Mountain Pose – Stand straight with your feet together. Pull in your stomach muscles as tight as you can and let your shoulders relax. Keep your legs strong but do not lock your knees. Breathe deeply and regularly in and out for ten breaths.

Strength Training – This activity is especially important for you to ensure you keep your muscles strong and healthy for the next phase of your life. You can do many strength training activities without weights, or for an extra challenge add some light hand weights.

Punching – This will strengthen your arms and shoulders and get your blood moving at the same time. Stand straight with your feet apart slightly wider than your shoulders. Keep your stomach firm. Punch straight out with one fist and then the other for at least twenty repetitions.

Squat – This activity is great for strengthening the bottom and the thighs. This will help you to sit down – not fall down – and be able to rise from a seated position with ease and grace. Stand with your feet as far apart as your hips are wide to provide a stable stance. Push your bottom backward as you bend your knees. Your knees should never go out front further than your toes, and try to keep your weight over your heels. If you feel more secure this activity can be done in front of a chair in case you lose your balance and inadvertently sit down.

Bridge – Lie on your back with your knees bent and your feet as far apart as your hips. Keep your feet flat on the floor. Pull in your stomach and lift your hips to make a bridge of your back. Hold this pose for ten seconds and try to do at least ten.

Cardiovascular/Aerobic – The purpose here is to engage in some activity that gets your heart pumping faster and your lungs expanding further. Swimming, walking, running, cycling, aerobics classes, dancing – all of these are great activities for getting the circulation going again. Just remember to begin slowly and pay attention to your body. In other words, if something hurts, stop. But make sure it is really hurt. There is a difference between 'Wow I'm really out of shape because I haven't walked anywhere in a while' and 'My knee really hurts when I do that'. And any time you are ever in doubt seek medical attention.

Seated Activities – The body will deteriorate if it is not used. Maybe you really want to engage in physical activities but you really can't stand up for long enough to do anything meaningful. You can sit down and do many activities that are designed to get you back into the routine of regular movement. Here are a few options for you:

Marching – sit tall in your chair with your feet flat on the floor and your legs bent at a ninety-degree angle. Lift one foot and then the other, as though you are marching in the chair. Raise the knee up in the air and keep the knee bent.

Shoulder Press – Sit tall in your chair. You can hold a set of light weights or simply make your hands into fists. If you do not own weights and do not want to buy any you can also use canned items or full water bottles. Raise your hands up into the air until your arms are straight and then lower them. Do these slowly so that your muscles will actually be doing the work.

Leg lifts – This activity will strengthen your quads, which is the muscle on the front of your leg. Strong quads are needed for walking upright. Sit tall in your chair with your knees bent at ninety degrees and your feet flat on the floor. Lift a foot up into the air and away from the chair slowly; let the muscle do the work. Hold the pose for five seconds and lower it. Repeat five times on each leg.

These are just a few of the activities that you can do to get yourself moving and help you in your weight loss and health goals. You are not too old to begin. You can find many routines on the internet so that you can use them alone in the privacy of your home. Remember to preview a routine before you pay for anything in case you do not like it. And many routines are offered free of charge. So do a bit of research and don't stop with one activity. Try to make your routine as varied as possible so that you will not get bored and soon you will have that body you want along with a healthier you.

Chapter 10:

Additional Things That Can Help

Yes, Keto is beneficial and yes, it has a lot of benefits, but it is no small thing and so, it must be approached with caution. Here are some tips you should keep in mind before embarking on Keto.

<u>Make use of recipes you can trust</u>

Keto involves a lot of meal planning and this single phase is where a lot of people get it wrong. Your meals are no longer allowed to be careless and you must note everything that goes into your mouth. If you are embarking on a Keto diet, you must use recipes you can trust. The recipes must be beneficial, safe, and delicious. Keto should not take out the enjoyment in your meals. Luckily, you have your hands on the best book for Keto aspirants under 50.

<u>You may need a doctor</u>

If you have had any issue with blood sugar, insulin levels or diabetes, consult your doctor before embarking on Keto. Do not make any dietary changes as large as Keto to your diet without first informing your doctor. He or she is in the best position to guide you properly. See your doctor.

<u>It will be hard at first</u>

Keto is no walk in the park. However, people continue on the path of Keto despite the initial difficulty because the results are evident after a short while. When you kick-start Keto, you may suffer from low blood sugar, sluggishness, and constipation, However, they will all wear off in a few days if you are religious about it.

Can Keto have side effects?

Yes. Keto can have side effects. Keto can have negative side effects if it is wrongly done. Keto cuts down on carbs and replaces them with fat. However, if the replacement is not adequately carried out, a lot of negative side effects may occur. This is why it is extremely important to begin the Keto diet armed with the right information and recipes which are all included in this book.

If you do not make use of quality meal plans and recipes, you'll lack nutrients that your body needs. With Keto, you must not lack proteins and so, your meals must be planned.

How to reach ketosis

Reaching the state of ketosis is not so straightforward for many people. In order to effectively reach ketosis, there are some steps you must take.

Eat the right food- Ketosis relies a lot on what you eat. To reach ketosis, you need to first cut down on the carbohydrates you take in. Secondly, you need to take in much more fats in your diets. However, you should just take in any fat, you should make sure to take in healthy fat. Taking in unhealthy fats can cause more harm than good.

Exercise- To efficiently reach ketosis, you should make sure to exercise. It doesn't have to be intensive, however, long walks, jugs, biking, and other exercises can help your body reach ketosis.

Try intermittent fasting- Some people combine intermittent fasting with ketosis. The reason is that, as you progress, your hunger pangs are reduced greatly and you will find intermittent fasting easy. In fact, even when you do not plan to, you'll find yourself doing it. It is definitely not compulsory but if you are making use of ketosis to lose weight, intermittent fasting is a great bonus.

Take lots of fruits and vegetables- Fruits and vegetables for snacks will keep your body healthy and help revitalize your skin.

Include coconut oil in your diet- Coconut is compulsory if you want to reach ketosis. Coconut oil contains healthy fat. It helps the body reach ketosis and contains four types of MCTs. It is one of the best tools for inducing ketosis. If you have never made use of coconut oil before, start slowly and increase your intake gradually.

<u>What are macros?</u>

'Macros' is short for macronutrients. These macronutrients are the important nutrients your body needs. These nutrients are-

Carbohydrates: In this group, we have sugars, fibers, and starches. Carbohydrates are broken down into glucose or blood sugar. Your body can then use it as energy or store it as glycogen in your liver or in your muscles.

Proteins: Proteins are found in fish, meat, eggs, and lentils such as beans. Proteins are necessary for a lot of functions such as cell signaling, the building of tissues, building of enzymes, as well as hormones. It is also necessary for various immune functions.

Fats: Fat is found in oils, butter, nuts, meat, fatty fish, and avocado. Fat is used for a lot of important things in the body. It helps maintain body temperature and produce hormones. It also helps the body absorb nutrients.

The Keto diet focuses on providing adequate levels of protein and substituting carbs for healthy fat.

Although some foods have the nutrients you need, they may also have a high level of carbs. This is why it is important to check the nutritional composition of any food before incorporating it into your diet

<u>Getting started with keto over 50</u>

There are various types of Keto diets. At 50 and above, you cannot just make use of the normal Keto diet. This is because at this age, each and everything you eat matters. You literally become what you eat and so, it is essential that you make use of the right variation of Keto.

You cannot make use of the traditional Keto diet as it is not suitable for older persons. Whatever Keto diet you'll be on must be suitable for your age and take into consideration that your body doesn't metabolize as fast as previously. It isn't what we want to hear, but it is what we need.

What not to eat when Ketoing:

Sugar

Starches and food high in carbohydrates

Too much fruit as it contains sugar when in large quantities.

Beer and Alcohol

Keto Diet for Below 50 VS Keto for Above 50

Those who are younger than 50 years of age find that they can stick to traditional Keto diets with no problems. They have schedules, cheat days, and other tools that help them. Missing a day or two does not have too serious repercussions as they can make up. However, one over 50, Ketoing has to be taken more seriously simply because it is harder to lose weight.

Due to the fact that it becomes harder to lose weight, a lot of over 50's have made Ketoing the 'rule' and not the exception. A careful study of this book will show that all the great recipes have been converted to Keto forms. Carbs were taken and replaced with fats and proteins are highly favored.

When 50 or above, your Keto diet must be followed religiously. This used to be a problem as most of the things we loved just involved a lot of carbs. Luckily, that is no longer the case. With the right recipe book, you will find it much easier to do without carbs.

Remember to run any dietary changes by your doctor.

Chapter 11: 21-Day Keto Meal Plan

Meal Plan	*Breakfast*	*Lunch*	*Dinner*	*Snacks*
DAY-1	Crispy Waffles	Super Salmon Parcel	Winter Comfort stew	Protein Rich Smoothie
DAY-2	Anti-Inflammatory Muffins	New England Salmon Pie	Ideal Cold Weather Stew	Morning Wake-Up Smoothie
DAY-3	Mini Crustless Quiches	Sweet & Sour Grouper	Weekend Dinner Stew	Blue Heaven Smoothie
DAY-4	French Baked Eggs	Aromatic Cod	Mexican Pork Stew	Dreamy Raspberry Smoothie
DAY-5	Zingy Scramble	Flavorsome Cod Bake	Hungarian Pork Stew	Sweet Holiday Smoothie
DAY-6	Potluck Lamb Salad	Wonderful Cod Platter	Yellow Chicken Soup	Fat-Flush Smoothie
DAY-7	Spring Supper Salad	Super-Simple Trout	Best Leftover Turkey Soup	2 Berries Smoothie
DAY-8	Chicken-of-Sea Salad	Classic Pork Tenderloin	Filling Beef Soup	Yummy Roasted Cauliflower
DAY-9	Vinegar Braised Cabbage	Signature Italian Pork Dish	Fabulous Beef Soup	Cheesy Cauliflower Mash
DAY-10	Green Veggies Curry	Flavor Packed Pork Loin	Warming Meatballs Soup	Buttered Broccoli
DAY-	Fuss-Free Veggies	Spiced Pork	Super Salmon	Great Side Dish

11	Bake	Tenderloin	Parcel	
DAY-12	4 Veggies Combo	Sticky Pork Ribs	New England Salmon Pie	Appealing Broccoli Mash
DAY-13	Midweek Veggie Supper	Valentine's Day Dinner	Sweet & Sour Grouper	Zesty Brussels Sprout
DAY-14	Buttery Veggies	South East Asian Steak Platter	Aromatic Cod	Simplest Yellow Squash
DAY-15	Best Tasting Kabobs	Pesto Flavored Steak	Flavorsome Cod Bake	Protein Rich Smoothie
DAY-16	Crispy Waffles	Flawless Grilled Steak	Wonderful Cod Platter	Morning Wake-Up Smoothie
DAY-17	Anti Inflammatory Muffins	Mongolian Beef	Super-Simple Trout	Blue Heaven Smoothie
DAY-18	Mini Crustless Quiches	Sicilian Steak Pinwheel	Winter Comfort stew	Dreamy Raspberry Smoothie
DAY-19	French Baked Eggs	American Beef Wellington	Ideal Cold Weather Stew	Sweet Holiday Smoothie
DAY-20	Zingy Scramble	Pastry-Free Beef Wellington	Weekend Dinner Stew	Fat-Flush Smoothie
DAY-21	Spring Supper Salad	New England Salmon Pie	Mexican Pork Stew	2 Berries Smoothie

Chapter 12:

Breakfast Recipes

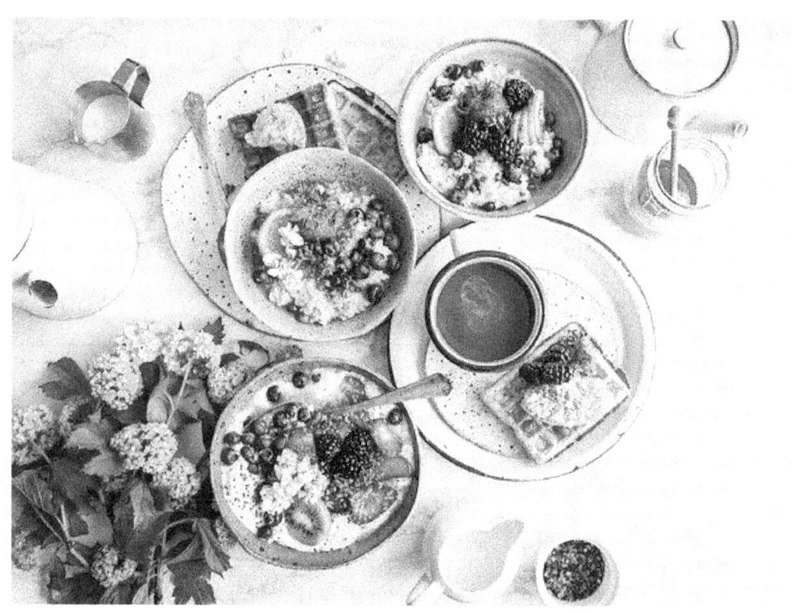

Crispy Waffles

Servings: 4

Cooking Time: 20 minutes

Preparation Time: 15 minutes

Ingredients: ½ C. super fine almond flour ½ tsp. Swerve ¼ tsp. organic baking powder

¼ tsp. baking soda ¼ tsp. ground cinnamon 1/8 tsp. ground cloves 1/8 tsp. ground nutmeg

¼ tsp. salt 2 organic eggs (whites and yolks separated) 2 tbsp. butter, melted

1 tsp. organic vanilla extract

Directions:

In a bowl, add the flour, Swerve, baking powder, baking soda, spices and salt and mix well.

In a second bowl, add the egg yolks, butter and vanilla and beat until well combined.

In a third small bowl, add the egg whites and beat until soft peaks form.

Add the egg yolks mixture into flour mixture and mix until well combined.

Gently, fold in the beaten egg whites.

Place ¼ of the mixture into preheated waffle iron and cook for about 4-5 minutes or until golden brown.

Repeat with the remaining mixture.

Serve warm.

Nutrition:

Calories: 167; Carbohydrates: 3.9g; Protein: 5.6g; Fat: 15g;

Sugar: 0.8g;

Sodium: 299mg; Fiber: 1.6g

Anti Inflammatory Muffins

Servings: 6

Cooking Time: 23 minutes

Preparation Time: 10 minutes

Ingredients: 2 C. almond flour ½ C. powdered Swerve 3 scoops turmeric tonic

1½ tsp. organic baking powder 3 organic eggs 1 C. mayonnaise ½ tsp. organic vanilla extract

Directions:

Preheat the oven to 350 degrees F. Line a 12 cups muffin tin with paper liners.

In a large bowl, add the flour, Swerve, turmeric tonic and baking powder and mix well.

Add the eggs, mayonnaise and vanilla extract and beat until well combined. Place the mixture into the prepared muffin cups evenly. Bake for about 20-23 minutes or until a toothpick inserted in the center comes out clean.

Remove the muffin tin from oven and place onto a wire rack to cool for about 10 minutes.

Carefully invert the muffins onto the wire rack to cool completely before serving.

Nutrition:

Calories: 489; Carbohydrates: 9.5g; Protein: 10.8g; Fat: 47.6g; Sugar: 1.9g; Sodium: 272mg;

Fiber: 4.1g

Mini Crustless Quiches

Servings: 6

Cooking Time: 30 minutes

Preparation Time: 15 minutes

Ingredients: 1 tsp. olive oil 1½ C. fresh mushrooms, chopped 1 scallion, chopped

1 tsp. garlic, mince 1 tsp. fresh rosemary, minced Freshly ground black pepper, to taste

1 (12.3-oz.) package lite firm silken tofu, drained   ¼ C. unsweetened almond milk

2 tbsp. Parmesan cheese, grated 1 tbsp. arrowroot starch 1 tsp. butter, softened

¼ tsp. ground turmeric

Directions:

Preheat the oven to 375 degrees F. Grease a 12 cups muffin tin.

In a nonstick skillet, heat the oil over medium heat and sauté the scallion and garlic for about 1 minute.

Add the mushrooms and sauté for about 5-7 minutes.

Stir in the rosemary and black pepper and remove from the heat

Set aside to cool slightly.

In a food processor, add the tofu and remaining ingredients and pulse until smooth.

Transfer the tofu mixture into a large bowl.

Fold in the mushroom mixture.

Place the mixture into the prepared muffin cups evenly.

10) Bake for about 20-22 minutes or until a toothpick inserted in the center comes out clean.

11) Remove the muffin pan from the oven and place onto a wire rack to cool for about 10 minutes.

12) Carefully, invert the muffins onto wire rack and serve warm.

Nutrition:

Calories: 77;

Carbohydrates: 5.3g;

Protein: 6.9g;

Fat: 3.7g;

Sugar: 1.9g;

Sodium: 52mg;

Fiber: 1g

French Baked Eggs

Servings: 4

Cooking Time: 12 minutes

Preparation Time: 10 minutes

Ingredients: 4 tbsp. half-and-half   4 organic eggs ½ oz. Gruyere cheese, shredded

Salt and freshly ground black pepper, to taste 4 tsp. fresh chives, minced

Directions:

Preheat the oven to 375 degrees F. Grease 4 ramekins.

In the bottom of each prepared ramekin, place 1 tbsp. of the heavy cream.

Carefully, crack 1 egg into each ramekin and sprinkle with the cheese, followed by salt, black pepper and chives.

Bake for about 8-12 minutes until the desired doneness of the eggs.

Serve hot.

Nutrition:

Calories: 97; Carbohydrates: 1g; Protein: 7.1g; Fat: 7.3g; Sugar: 0.4g; Sodium: 118mg; Fiber: 0g

Zingy Scramble

Servings: 4

Cooking Time: 6 minutes

Preparation Time: 10 minutes

Ingredients: 2 tbsp. unsalted butter 1 tomato, chopped finely 1 scallion, chopped finely

2 pickled jalapeños, chopped finely 6 organic eggs, beaten 3 oz. Colby jack cheese, shredded

Salt and freshly ground black pepper, to taste

Directions:

In a large frying pan, melt the butter over medium-high heat and cook the tomato, scallion and jalapeños for about 3-4 minutes, stirring frequently.

Add the eggs and cook for about 2 minutes, stirring continuously.

Stir in the cheese, salt and black pepper and remove from the heat.

Serve hot.

Nutrition:

Calories: 235; Carbohydrates: 2.7g; Protein: 13.2g; Fat: 19.2g; Sugar: 1.3g;

Sodium: 492mg; Fiber: 0.6g

No-Cooking Breakfast Bowl

Servings: 1

Cooking Time: 0 minutes

Preparation Time: 10 minutes

Ingredients: 2/3 C. frozen raspberries 1/3 C. frozen cauliflower rice

1 medium avocado, peeled, pitted and chopped roughly

1 scoop unsweetened vanilla protein powder 1 tsp. beet powder ¼ C. unsweetened almond milk

Directions:

In a high-speed blender, add all the ingredients and pulse until smooth.

Transfer into 2 serving bowls and serve with your favorite topping.

Nutrition:

Calories: 125;

Carbohydrates: 8.9g;

Protein: 14.3g; Fat: 3.8g;

Sugar: 2.2g;

Sodium: 165mg; Fiber: 4.9g

Super Food Smoothie Bowl

Servings: 2

Preparation Time: 10 minutes

Ingredients:

2 C. fresh spinach

1 medium avocado, peeled, pitted and chopped roughly

1 scoop unflavored collagen powder

1 scoop MCT oil powder

¼ C. Erythritol

2 tbsp. fresh lemon juice

1 C. unsweetened almond milk

¼ C. Ice cubes

Directions:

In a high-speed blender, add all the ingredients and pulse until smooth.

Transfer into 2 serving bowls and serve with your favorite topping.

Nutrition:

Calories: 304; Carbohydrates: 12g; Protein: 17.6g; Fat: 22.4g; Sugar: 1g; Sodium: 146mg; Fiber: 8g

Nutty Textured Porridge

Servings: 5

Cooking Time: 35 minutes

Preparation Time: 15 minutes

Ingredients: ½ C. pecans ½ C. walnuts ¼ C. sunflower seeds ¼ C. chia seeds

¼ C. unsweetened coconut flakes 4 C. unsweetened almond milk ½ tsp. ground cinnamon

¼ tsp. ground ginger 1 tsp. stevia powder 1 tbsp. butter

Directions:

In a food processor, place the pecans, walnuts and sunflower seeds and pulse until a crumbly mixture is formed.

In a large pan, add the nuts mixture, chia seeds, coconut flakes, almond milk, spices and stevia powder over medium heat and bring to a gentle simmer, stirring frequently.

Reduce the heat to low and simmer for about 20-30 minutes, stirring frequently.

Remove from the heat and serve hot with the topping of butter.

Nutrition:

Calories: 269; Carbohydrates: 8.6g; Protein: 7.1g;

Fat: 25.9g; Sugar: 0.8g; Sodium: 161mg; Fiber: 5.7g

Chapter 13:

Lunch Recipes

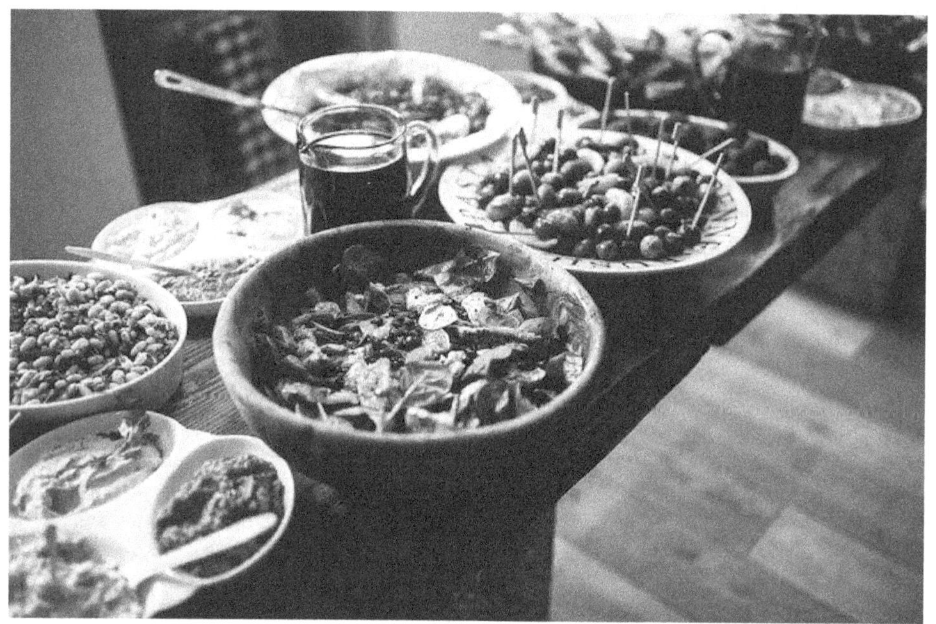

Bacon Burger Cabbage Stir Fry

Preparation time: 10 minutes

Cooking time: 20 minutes

Servings: 10

Ingredients: Ground beef (1 lb.) Bacon (1 lb.) Small onion (1) Minced cloves of garlic (3)

Cabbage (1 lb./1 small head)

Directions: Dice the bacon and onion. Combine the beef and bacon in a wok or large skillet. Prepare it until done and store it in a bowl to keep warm. Mince the onion and garlic. Toss both into the hot grease. Slice and toss in the cabbage and stir-fry until wilted. Blend in the meat and combine. Sprinkle with pepper and salt as desired.

Nutrition:

Net Carbohydrates: 4.5 grams Protein Counts: 32 grams Total Fats: 22 grams Calories: 357

Bacon Cheeseburger

Preparation time: 15 minutes

Cooking time: 30 minutes

Servings: 12

Ingredients: Low-sodium bacon (16 oz. pkg.) Ground beef (3 lb.) Eggs (2)

Medium chopped onion (half of 1) Shredded cheddar cheese (8 oz.)

Directions: Fry the bacon and chop it to bits. Shred the cheese and dice the onion. Combine the mixture with the beef and blend in the whisked eggs. Prepare 24 burgers and grill them the way you like them. You can make a double-decker since they are small. If you like a bigger burger, you can make 12 burgers as a single-decker.

Nutrition: Net Carbohydrates: 0.8 grams Protein Counts: 27 grams Total Fats: 41 grams

Calories: 489

Cauliflower Mac & Cheese

Preparation time: 15 minutes

Cooking time: 20 minutes

Servings: 4

Ingredients:

Cauliflower (1 head) Butter (3 tbsp.) Unsweetened almond milk (.25 cup)

Heavy cream (.25 cup) Cheddar cheese (1 cup)

Directions:

Use a sharp knife to slice the cauliflower into small florets. Shred the cheese. Prepare the oven to reach 450° Fahrenheit. Cover a baking pan with a layer of parchment baking paper or foil.

Add two tablespoons of the butter to a pan and melt. Add the florets, butter, salt, and pepper together. Place the cauliflower on the baking pan and roast 10 to 15 minutes.

Warm up the rest of the butter, milk, heavy cream, and cheese in the microwave or double boiler. Pour the cheese over the cauliflower and serve.

Nutrition:

Net Carbohydrates: 7 grams

Protein Counts: 11 grams Total Fats: 23 grams Calories: 294

Mushroom & Cauliflower Risotto

Preparation time: 5 minutes

Cooking time: 10 minutes

Servings: 4

Ingredients:

Grated head of cauliflower (1)

Vegetable stock (1 cup)

Chopped mushrooms (9 oz.)

Butter (2 tbsp.)

Coconut cream (1 cup)

Directions:

Pour the stock in a saucepan. Boil and set aside. Prepare a skillet with butter and saute the mushrooms until golden.

Grate and stir in the cauliflower and stock. Simmer and add the cream, cooking until the cauliflower is al dente. Serve.

Nutrition:

Net Carbohydrates: 4 grams Protein Counts: 1 gram Total Fats: 17 grams Calories: 186

Pita Pizza

Preparation time: 15 minutes

Cooking time: 10 minutes

Servings: 2

Ingredients:

Marinara sauce (.5 cup) Low-carb pita (1) Cheddar cheese (2 oz.)

Pepperoni (14 slices) Roasted red peppers (1 oz.)

Directions:

Program the oven temperature setting to 450° Fahrenheit.

Slice the pita in half and place onto a foil-lined baking tray. Rub with a bit of oil and toast for one to two minutes.

Pour the sauce over the bread. Sprinkle using the cheese and other toppings. Bake until the cheese melts (5 min.). Cool thoroughly.

Nutrition:

Net Carbohydrates: 4 grams

Protein Counts: 13 grams

Total Fats: 19 grams

Calories: 250

Skillet Cabbage Tacos

Preparation time: 10 minutes

Cooking time: 15 minutes

Servings: 4

Ingredients:

Ground beef (1 lb.) Salsa - ex. Pace Organic (.5 cup)

Shredded cabbage (2 cups) Chili powder (2 tsp.) Shredded cheese (.75 cup)

Directions:

Brown the beef and drain the fat. Pour in the salsa, cabbage, and seasoning.

Cover and lower the heat. Simmer for 10 to 12 minutes using the medium heat temperature setting.

When the cabbage has softened, remove it from the heat and mix in the cheese.

Top it off using your favorite toppings, such as green onions or sour cream, and serve.

Nutrition:

Net Carbohydrates: 4 grams

Protein Counts: 30 grams Total Fats: 21 grams Calories: 325

Taco Casserole

Preparation time: 10 minutes

Cooking time: 20 minutes

Servings: 8

Ingredients:

Ground turkey or beef (1.5 to 2 lb.)

Taco seasoning (2 tbsp.) Shredded cheddar cheese (8 oz.)

Salsa (1 cup) Cottage cheese (16 oz.)

Directions:

Heat the oven to reach 400° Fahrenheit.

Combine the taco seasoning and ground meat in a casserole dish. Bake it for 20 minutes.

Combine the salsa and both kinds of cheese. Set aside for now.

Carefully transfer the casserole dish from the oven. Drain away the cooking juices from the meat.

Break the meat into small pieces and mash with a potato masher or fork.

Sprinkle with cheese. Bake in the oven for 15 to 20 more minutes until the top is browned.

Nutrition:

Net Carbohydrates: 6 grams Protein Counts: 45 grams Total Fats: 18 grams Calories: 367

Creamy Chicken Salad

Preparation time: 10 minutes

Cooking time: 30 minutes

Servings: 4

Ingredients: Chicken Breast - 1 Lb. Avocado - 2 Garlic Cloves - 2, Minced Lime Juice - 3 T.

Onion - .33 C., Minced Jalapeno Pepper - 1, Minced Salt - Dash Cilantro - 1 T. Pepper - Dash

Directions

If you like traditional chicken salad, this is an excellent alternative to help provide healthier fats along with a good chunk of protein. You will want to start this recipe off my prepping the stove to 400. As this warms up, get out your cooking sheet and line it with paper or foil. Next, it is time to get out the chicken. Go ahead and layer the chicken breast up with some olive oil before seasoning to your liking. I generally use salt and pepper, but feel free to use anything like garlic or onion powder! When the chicken is all set, you will want to line them along the surface of your cooking sheet and pop it into the oven for about twenty minutes. By the end of twenty minutes, the chicken should be cooked through and can be taken out of the oven for chilling. Once cool enough to handle, you will want to either dice or shred your chicken, dependent upon how you like your chicken salad. Now that your chicken is all cooked, it is time to assemble your salad! You can begin this process by adding everything into a bowl and mashing down the avocado. Once your ingredients are mended to your liking, sprinkle some salt over the top and serve immediately. Whether you like your chicken salad straight out of the bowl or in a low-carb wrap, it can be enjoyed in a number of different ways!

Nutrition: Fats: 20g Carbs: 4g Proteins: 25g

Spicy Keto Chicken Wings

Preparation time: 20 minutes

Cooking time: 30 minutes

Servings: 4

Ingredients:

Chicken Wings - 2 Lbs. Cajun Spice - 1 t.

Smoked Paprika - 2 t.

Turmeric - .50 t.

Salt - Dash

Baking Powder - 2 t.

Pepper - Dash

Directions:

When you first begin the Ketogenic Diet, you may find that you won't be eating the traditional foods that may have made up a majority of your diet in the past. While this is a good thing for your health, you may feel you are missing out! The good news is that there are delicious alternatives that aren't lacking in flavor! To start this recipe, you'll want to prep the stove to 400.

As this heats up, you will want to take some time to dry your chicken wings with a paper towel. This will help remove any excess moisture and get you some nice, crispy wings!

When you are all set, take out a mixing bowl and place all of the seasonings along with the baking powder. If you feel like it, you can adjust the seasoning levels however you would like. Once these are set, go ahead and throw the chicken wings in and coat evenly. If you have one, you'll want to place the wings on a wire rack that is placed over your baking tray. If not, you can just lay them across the baking sheet.

Now that your chicken wings are set, you are going to pop them into the stove for thirty minutes. By the end of this time, the tops of the wings should be crispy. If they are, take them out from the oven and flip them so that you can bake the other side. You will want to cook these for an additional thirty minutes.

Finally, take the tray from the oven and allow to cool slightly before serving up your spiced keto wings. For additional flavor, serve with any of your favorite, keto-friendly dipping sauce.

Nutrition:

Fats: 7g

Carbs: 1g

Proteins: 60g

Cilantro and Lime Creamed Chicken

Preparation time: 10 minutes

Cooking time: 20 minutes

Servings: 4

Ingredients: Chicken Breast - 4 Pieces Red Pepper Flakes - 1 t. Cilantro - 1 T. Salt - Dash

Lime Juice - 2 T. Chicken Broth - 1 C. Onion - .25 C., Chopped Olive Oil - 1 T.

Heavy Cream - .50 C. Pepper - Dash

Directions: If you are looking for a dish that is a bit different, this recipe is going to be perfect for you. Between the cilantro and the lime, this dish offers a fresh twist on traditional chicken. Many people feel that in order to lose weight, they need to give up flavor, but on the Ketogenic Diet, that is simply not the case! To begin this recipe, you will want to get out your cooking skillet and place it over a moderate temperature. As the skillet heats, go ahead and season the chicken breast according to your taste. For this particular recipe, you will want to consider using the seasonings provided in the list above, but feel free to adjust levels to your own taste. Once seasoned to your liking, throw the chicken into the skillet and cook for about eight minutes on each side. When the chicken is cooked through, take it out of the pan and place to the side. Next, you are going to add the onion into the hot pan and cook them for a minute before also adding in the cilantro, pepper flakes, lime juice, and the chicken broth. If you don't have chicken broth on hand, feel free to use water. Once these items are in place, bring to a boil for ten minutes. Last-minute, you are going to whisk in your heavy cream and add in the chicken so that it can be coated in the sauce you just made. For extra flavor, add in some more cilantro, and then your chicken can be served by itself or with a keto-friendly vegetable!

Nutrition: Fats: 20g Carbs: 6g Proteins: 30g

Cheesy Ham Quiche

Preparation time: 10 minutes

Cooking time: 30 minutes

Servings: 6

Ingredients: Eggs - 8 Zucchini - 1 C., Shredded eavy Cream - .50 C. Ham - 1 C., Diced

Mustard - 1 t. Salt - Dash

Directions:

Unlike traditional quiche, this version is crustless! Because there is no crust, this recipe offers a low-carb option for those who are still looking to make a savory meal for breakfast or lunch. For this recipe, you can start off by prepping your stove to 375 and getting out a pie plate for your quiche. Next, it is time to prep the zucchini. First, you will want to go ahead and shred it into small pieces. Once this is complete, take a paper towel and gently squeeze out the excess moisture. This will help avoid a soggy quiche. When the step from above is complete, you will want to place the zucchini into your pie plate along with the cooked ham pieces and your cheese. Once these items are in place, you will want to whisk the seasonings, cream, and eggs together before pouring it over the top. Now that your quiche is set, you are going to pop the dish into your stove for about forty minutes. By the end of this time, the egg should be cooked through, and you will be able to insert a knife into the center and have it come out clean. If the quiche is cooked to your liking, take the dish from the oven and allow it to chill slightly before slicing and serving.

Nutrition: Fats: 25g Carbs: 2g Proteins: 20g

Loaded Cauliflower Rice

Preparation time: 10 minutes

Cooking time: 20 minutes

Servings: 4

Ingredients: Cauliflower - 1 Head   Cheddar Cheese - 1 C.   Bacon - 1 Lb.

Chives - .50 C. Salt - Dash

Directions:

Sometimes, you just want something basic for lunch. This loaded cauliflower rice is fairly easy to make and only requires a handful of ingredients! The first step of this recipe is going to be ricing your cauliflower. You can choose to do this by hand, or you can purchase cauliflower rice in the frozen section.

Next, you will want to take several moments to cook your bacon. You can complete this task by heating a grilling pan over a moderate temperature and cook the bacon for four or five minutes on either side. I like my bacon crispy, but that is completely up to you!

When you are set, you are going to place your cauliflower rice into a microwave-safe bowl and sprinkle your shredded cheese over the top. When this is set, go ahead and pop the bowl into the microwave for a minute and allow for the rice to cook through and the cheese to melt. Once the step from above is complete, top the dish off with your bacon pieces and season to your liking. Just like that, lunch will be ready for you!

Nutrition:

Fats: 10g   Carbs: 5g   Proteins: 5g

Super Herbed Fish

Preparation time: 8-10 minutes

Cooking time: 6 minutes

Servings: 1

Ingredients: 1 tablespoon chopped basil   2 teaspoons lime zest   1 tablespoon lime juice

1 tablespoon olive oil 1 4-ounce fish fillet 1 rosemary sprig 1 thyme sprig 1 ½ cups water

1 teaspoon Dijon mustard   ¼ teaspoon garlic powder   Pinch of salt   Pinch of pepper

Directions:

Season the fish with salt and paper. Arrange on a piece of parchment paper and sprinkle with zest. Whisk together the oil, juice, and mustard in a mixing bowl and brush over. Top with the herbs. Wrap the fish with the parchment paper. Wrap the wrapped fish in an aluminum foil. Arrange Instant Pot over a dry platform in your kitchen. Open its top lid and switch it on. In the pot, pour water. Arrange a trivet or steamer basket inside that came with Instant Pot. Now place/arrange the foil over the trivet/basket. Close the lid to create a locked chamber; make sure that safety valve is in locking position. Find and press "MANUAL" cooking function; timer to 5 minutes with default "HIGH" pressure mode. Allow the pressure to build to cook the ingredients. After cooking time is over press "CANCEL" setting. Find and press "QPR" cooking function. This setting is for quick release of inside pressure. Slowly open the lid, take out the cooked recipe in serving plates or serving bowls, and enjoy the keto recipe.

Nutrition: Calories - 246 Fat – 9g Saturated Fat – 1g Trans Fat – 0g Carbohydrates – 1g

Fiber – 0.5g Sodium – 86mg   Protein – 28g

Chapter 14:

Dinner Recipes

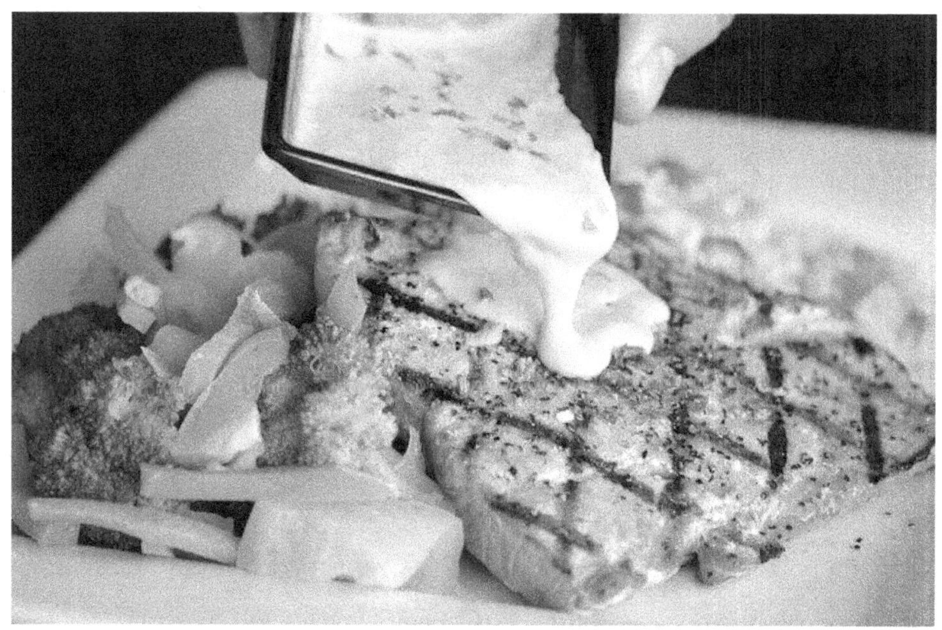

Chicken Pan with Veggies and Pesto

Preparation time: 10 minutes

Cooking time: 20 minutes

Servings: 4

Ingredients: 2 Tbsp olive oil 1 pound chicken thighs, boneless, skinless, sliced into strips

¾ cup oil-packed sun-dried tomatoes, chopped 1 pound asparagus ends

¼ cup basil pesto 1 cup cherry tomatoes, red and yellow, halved Salt, to taste

Directions:

1.   Heat olive oil in a frying pan over medium-high heat.

2.   Put salt on the chicken slices and the put into a skillet, add the sun-dried tomatoes and fry for 5-10 minutes. Remove the chicken slices and season with salt. Add asparagus to the skillet. Cook for additional 5-10 minutes.

3.   Place the chicken back in the skillet, pour in the pesto and whisk. Fry for 1-2 minutes. Remove from the heat. Add the halved cherry tomatoes and pesto. Stir well and serve.

Nutrition :

Carbohydrates – 12 g Fat – 32 g Protein – 2 g Calories – 423

Cabbage Soup with Beef

Prep time: 15 minutes

Cooking time: 20 minutes

Servings: 4

Ingredients: 2 Tbsp olive oil 1 medium onion, chopped 1 pound fillet steak, cut into pieces

½ stalk celery, chopped 1 carrot, peeled and diced ½ head small green cabbage, cut into pieces

2 cloves garlic, minced 4 cups beef broth 2 Tbsp fresh parsley, chopped 1 tsp dried thyme

1 tsp dried rosemary 1 tsp garlic powder Salt and black pepper, to taste

Directions:

1.   Heat oil in a pot (use medium heat). Add the beef and cook until it is browned. Put the onion into the pot and boil for 3-4 minutes.

2.   Add the celery and carrot. Stir well and cook for about 3-4 minutes. Add the cabbage and boil until it starts softening. Add garlic and simmer for about 1 minute.

3.   Pour the broth into the pot. Add the parsley and garlic powder. Mix thoroughly and reduce heat to medium-low.

4.   Cook for 10-15 minutes.

Nutrition : Carbohydrates – 4 g Fat – 11 g Protein – 12 g Calories –177

Cauliflower Rice Soup with Chicken

Prep time: 10 minutes

Cooking time: 1 hour

Servings: 5

Ingredients: 2½ pounds chicken breasts, boneless and skinless

8 Tbsp butter ¼ cup celery, chopped ½ cup onion, chopped

4 cloves garlic, minced 2 12-ounce packages steamed cauliflower rice

1 Tbsp parsley, chopped 2 tsp poultry seasoning ½ cup carrot, grated

¾ tsp rosemary

1 tsp salt

¾ tsp pepper

4 ounces cream cheese

4¾ cup chicken broth

Directions:

1.   Put shredded chicken breasts into a saucepan and pour in the chicken broth. Add salt and pepper. Cook for 1 hour.

2.   In another pot, melt the butter. Add the onion, garlic, and celery. Saute until the mix is translucent. Add the riced cauliflower, rosemary, and carrot. Mix and cook for 7 minutes.

3.   Add the chicken breasts and broth to the cauliflower mix. Put the lid on and simmer for 15 minutes.

Nutrition :

Carbohydrates – 6 g

Fat – 30 g

Protein – 27 g

Calories –415

Quick Pumpkin Soup

Prep time: 10 minutes

Cooking time: 20 minutes

Servings: 4-6

Ingredients: 1 cup coconut milk 2 cups chicken broth 6 cups baked pumpkin 1 tsp garlic powder

1 tsp ground cinnamon 1 tsp dried ginger 1 tsp nutmeg 1 tsp paprika Salt and pepper, to taste

Sour cream or coconut yogurt, for topping Pumpkin seeds, toasted, for topping

Directions:

1.   Combine the coconut milk, broth, baked pumpkin, and spices in a soup pan (use medium heat). Stir occasionally and simmer for 15 minutes.

2.   With an immersion blender, blend the soup mix for 1 minute.

3.   Top with sour cream or coconut yogurt and pumpkin seeds.

Nutrition :

Carbohydrates – 8.1 g

Fat – 9.8 g Protein – 3.1 g Calories – 123

Fresh Avocado Soup

Prep time: 5 minutes

Cooking time: 10 minutes

Servings: 2

Ingredients:

1 ripe avocado

2 romaine lettuce leaves, washed and chopped

1 cup coconut milk, chilled

1 Tbsp lime juice

20 fresh mint leaves

Salt, to taste

Directions:

1.   Mix all your ingredients thoroughly in a blender .

2.   Chill in the fridge for 5-10 minutes.

Nutrition :

Carbohydrates – 12 g Fat – 26 g Protein – 4 g Calories – 280

Creamy Garlic Chicken

Prep time: 5 minutes

Cooking time: 15 minutes

Servings: 4

Ingredients: 4 chicken breasts, finely sliced 1 tsp garlic powder 1 tsp paprika 2 Tbsp butter

1 tsp salt 1 cup heavy cream ½ cup sun-dried tomatoes 2 cloves garlic, minced

1 cup spinach, chopped

Directions:

1.   Blend the paprika, garlic powder, and salt and sprinkle over both sides of the chicken.

2.   Melt the butter in a frying pan (choose medium heat). Add the chicken breast and fry for 5 minutes each side. Set aside.

3.   Add the heavy cream, sun-dried tomatoes, and garlic to the pan and whisk well to combine. Cook for 2 minutes. Add spinach and saute for an additional 3 minutes. Return the chicken to the pan and cover with the sauce.

Nutrition :

Carbohydrates – 12 g Fat – 26 g Protein – 4 g Calories – 280

Cauliflower Cheesecake

Prep time: 20 minutes

Cooking time: 30 minutes

Servings: 6

Ingredients: 1 head cauliflower, cut into florets ⅔ cup sour cream 4 oz cream cheese, softened

1½ cup cheddar cheese, shredded 6 pieces bacon, cooked and chopped 1 tsp salt

½ tsp black pepper ¼ cup green onion, chopped ¼ tsp garlic powder

Directions:

1.   Preheat the oven to 350°F.

2.   Boil the cauliflower florets for 5 minutes.

3.   In a separate bowl combine the cream cheese and sour cream. Mix well and add the cheddar cheese, bacon pieces, green onion, salt, pepper, and garlic powder. Put the cauliflower florets into the bowl and combine with the sauce.

4.   Put the cauliflower mix on the baking tray and bake for 15-20 minutes.

Nutrition :

Carbohydrates – 8 g

Fat – 26 g Protein –15 g Calories – 320

Chinese Pork Bowl

Prep time: 5 minutes

Cooking time: 15 minutes

Servings: 4

Ingredients: Salt and ground black pepper, to taste

1¼ pounds pork belly, cut into bite-size pieces 2 Tbsp tamari soy sauce

1 Tbsp rice vinegar 2 cloves garlic, smashed 3 oz butter

1 pound Brussels sprouts, rinsed, trimmed, halved or quartered ½ leek, chopped

Directions:

1.   Fry the pork over medium-high heat until it is starting to turn golden brown.

2.   Combine the garlic cloves, butter, and brussel sprouts. Add to the pan, whisk well and cook until the sprouts turn golden brown.

3.   Stir the soy sauce and rice vinegar together and pour the sauce into the pan.

4.   Sprinkle with salt and pepper.

5.   Top with chopped leek.

Nutrition :

Carbohydrates – 7 g Fat – 97 g Protein – 19 g Calories – 993

Turkey-Pepper Mix

Prep time: 20 minutes

Cooking time: 0 minutes

Servings: 1

Ingredients: 1 pound turkey tenderloin, cut in thin steaks 1 tsp salt, divided

2 Tbsp extra-virgin olive oil, divided ½ sweet onion, sliced 1 red bell pepper, cut into strips

1 yellow bell pepper, cut into strips ½ tsp Italian seasoning ¼ tsp ground black pepper

2 tsp red wine vinegar 1 14-ounces can crushed tomatoes, roasted Fresh parsley Basil

Directions:

1.   Sprinkle ½ tsp salt on your turkey. Pour 1 Tbsp oil into the pan and heat it. Add the turkey steaks and cook for 1-3 minutes per side. Set aside.

2.   Put the onion, bell peppers, and the remaining salt to the pan and cook for 7 minutes, stirring all the time. Sprinkle with Italian seasoning and add black pepper. Cook for 30 seconds. Add the tomatoes and vinegar and fry the mix for about 20 seconds.

3.   Return the turkey to the pan and pour the sauce over it. Simmer for 2-3 minutes.

4.   Top with chopped parsley and basil.

Nutrition :

Carbohydrates – 11 g Fat – 8 g Protein –30 g Calories – 230

Shrimp Scampi with Garlic

Prep time: 5 minutes

Cooking time: 10 minutes

Servings: 4

Ingredients: ¼ cup parsley, chopped

1 pound shrimp 3 Tbsp olive oil 1 bulb shallot, sliced 4 cloves garlic, minced ½ cup Pinot Grigio

4 Tbsp salted butter 1 Tbsp lemon juice ½ tsp sea salt ¼ tsp black pepper ¼ tsp red pepper flakes

Directions:

1.   Pour the olive oil into the previously heated frying pan. Add the garlic and shallots and fry for about 2 minutes.

2.   Combine the Pinot Grigio, salted butter, and lemon juice. Pour this mix into the pan and cook for 5 minutes.

3.   Put the parsley, black pepper, red pepper flakes, and sea salt into the pan and whisk well.

4.   Add the shrimp and fry until they are pink (about 3 minutes).

Nutrition :

Carbohydrates – 7 g Fat – 7 g Protein – 32 g Calories – 344

Simple Tuna Salad

Prep time: 5 minutes

Cooking time: 0 minutes

Servings: 4

Ingredients:

10 oz canned tuna, drained 1 avocado, chopped 1 rib celery, chopped 2 cloves fresh garlic, minced

3 Tbsp mayonnaise 1 red onion, chopped Tbsp lemon juice 8 sprigs parsley

¼ cucumber, chopped Salt and pepper, to taste

Directions:

1.   Divide the parsley into two halves.

2.   Mix all the ingredients except half of the parsley in a separate bowl. Stir well.

3.   Add salt and pepper to taste.

4.   Top with the remaining parsley.

Nutrition :

Carbohydrates – 1.7 g Fat – 16.3 g Protein – 13.9 g Calories – 225

Chapter 15:

Vegetables Recipes

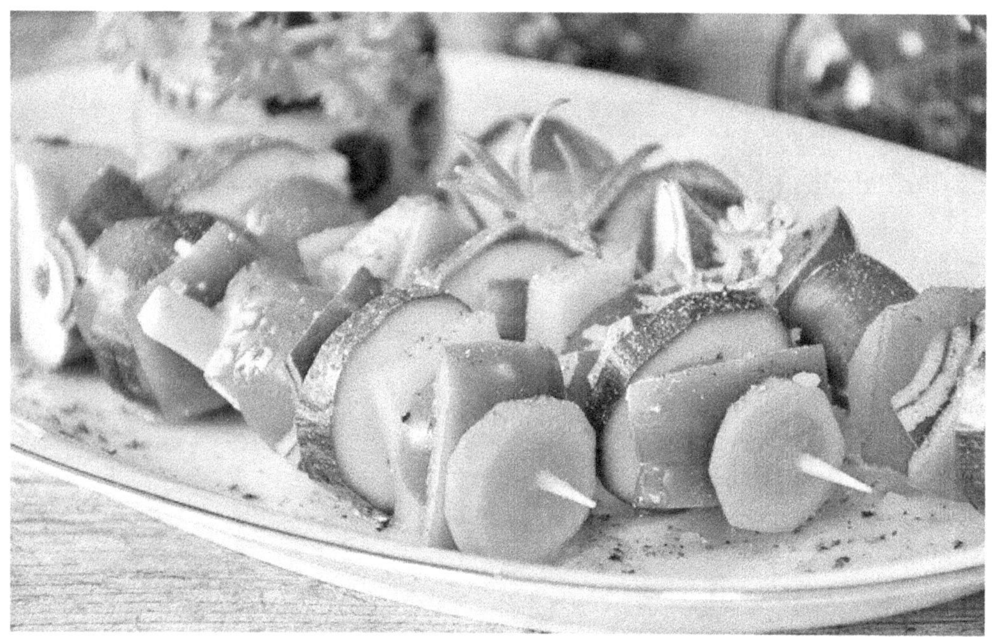

Scrumptious Cauliflower Casserole

Servings: 4

Cooking Time: 35 minutes

Preparation Time: 15 minutes

Ingredients: 1 large head cauliflower, cut into florets 2 tbsp. butter 2 oz. cream cheese, softened

1¼ C. sharp cheddar cheese, shredded and divided 1 C. heavy cream

Salt and freshly ground black pepper, to taste ¼ C. scallion, chopped and divided

Directions:

Preheat the oven to 350 0 F.

In a large pan of boiling water, add the cauliflower florets and cook for about 2 minutes.

Drain cauliflower and keep aside.

For cheese sauce: in a medium pan, add butter over medium-low heat and cook until just melted.

Add cream cheese, 1 C. of cheddar cheese, heavy cream, salt and black pepper and cook until melted and smooth, stirring continuously.

Remove from heat and keep aside to cool slightly.

In a baking dish, place cauliflower florets, cheese sauce, and 3 tbsp. of scallion and stir to combine well.

Sprinkle with remaining cheddar cheese and scallion.

Bake for about 30 minutes.

Remove the casserole dish from oven and set aside for about 5-10 minutes before serving.

Cut into 4 equal-sized portions and serve.

Nutrition:

Calories: 365; Carbohydrates: 5.6g; Protein: 12g; Fat: 33.6g; Sugar: 3g; Sodium: 373mg;

Fiber: 1.8g

Relatively Flavored Gratin

Servings: 8

Cooking Time: 46 minutes

Preparation Time: 15 minutes

Ingredients: ½ C. heavy whipping cream 2 tbsp. butter ½ tsp. garlic powder ¼ tsp. xanthan gum

4 C. zucchini, sliced 1 small yellow onion, thinly sliced

Salt and freshly ground black pepper, to taste 1½ C. pepper jack cheese, shredded

Directions:

Preheat the oven to 375 0 F and grease a 9×9-inch baking dish. In a microwave-safe dish, place the heavy whipping cream, butter, garlic powder, and xanthan gum and microwave for about 1 minute. Remove from microwave and beat the mixture until smooth. Arrange 1/3 of zucchini and onion slices in the bottom of prepared baking dish and sprinkle with some salt, black pepper and ½ C. of pepper jack cheese. Repeat the layers twice. Now, place the cream mixture on top evenly. Bake for about 45 minutes or until the top is golden brown. Remove the baking dish from oven and set aside for about 5-10 minutes before serving. Cut into 8 equal-sized portions and serve.

Nutrition:

Calories: 140; Carbohydrates: 3.9g; Protein: 5.5g; Fat: 11.8g; Sugar: 1.4g; Sodium: 242mg;

Fiber: 0.9g

Thanksgiving Veggie Meal

Servings: 6

Cooking Time: 30 minutes

Preparation Time: 20 minutes

Ingredients:

For Onion Slices:

½ C. yellow onion, sliced very thinly ¼ C. almond flour 1/8 tsp. garlic powder

Salt and freshly ground black pepper, to taste

For Casserole:

1 lb. fresh green beans, trimmed 1 tbsp. olive oil 8 oz. fresh cremini mushrooms, sliced

½ C. yellow onion, thinly sliced 1/8 tsp. garlic powder

Salt and freshly ground black pepper, to taste 1 tsp. fresh thyme, chopped

½ C. homemade vegetable broth ½ C. sour cream

Directions:

Preheat the oven to 350 0 F.

For onion slices: in a bowl, place all the ingredients and toss to coat well.

Arrange the onion slices onto a large baking sheet in a single layer.

In a pan of salted boiling water, add the green beans and cook for about 5 minutes.

Drain the green beans and transfer into a bowl of ice water.

Again, drain well and transfer into a large bowl.

In a large skillet, heat the oil over medium-high heat and sauté the mushrooms, onion, garlic powder, salt and black pepper for about 2-3 minutes.

Stir in the thyme, and broth and cook for about 3-5 minutes or until all the liquid is absorbed.

Remove from heat and transfer the mushroom mixture into the bowl with green beans.

Add the sour cream and stir to combine well.

Transfer the mixture into a 10-inch casserole dish.

Place the casserole dish and baking sheet of onion slices into the oven.

Bake for about 15-17 minutes.

Remove the baking dish from oven and let it cool for about 5 minutes before serving.

Top the casserole evenly with crispy onion slices.

Cut into 6 equal-sized portions and serve.

Nutrition:

Calories: 134; Carbohydrates: 10g; Protein: 4.6g; Fat: 8.8g; Sugar: 2.6g; Sodium: 110mg;

Fiber: 3.8g

Loaded Squash Casserole

Servings: 8

Cooking Time: 55 minutes

Preparation Time: 15 minutes

Ingredients: 2 tbsp. olive oil 1 small yellow onion, chopped 3 summer squashes, sliced

4 organic eggs, beaten 3 C. cheddar cheese, shredded and divided

2 tbsp. unsweetened almond milk 2-3 tbsp. almond flour 2 tbsp. Erythritol

Salt and freshly ground black pepper, to taste 1/3 C. unsalted butter, melted

Directions:

Preheat the oven to 375 0 F. In a large skillet, heat the oil over medium heat and cook the onion and squash for about 8-10 minutes, stirring occasionally. Remove from the heat. Place the eggs, 1 C. of cheddar cheese, almond milk, almond flour, Erythritol, salt and black pepper in a large bowl and mix until well combined. Add the squash mixture, and butter and stir to combine. Transfer the mixture into a large casserole dish and sprinkle with the remaining cheddar cheese. Bake for about 35-45 minutes. Remove the casserole dish from oven and set aside for about 5-10 minutes before serving. Cut into 8 equal-sized portions and serve.

Nutrition:

Calories: 383; Carbohydrates: 4.4g; Protein: 14.8g; Fat: 28.4g; Sugar: 2g;

Sodium: 379mg; Fiber: 1.2g

Meatless Cabbage Rolls

Servings: 8,

Cooking Time: 25 minutes,

Preparation Time: 25 minutes

Ingredients:

For Filling:

1½ C. fresh button mushrooms, chopped 3¼ C. zucchini, chopped

1 C. red bell pepper, seeded and chopped 1 C. green bell pepper, seeded and chopped

½ tsp. dried thyme, crushed ½ tsp. dried marjoram, crushed ½ tsp. dried basil, crushed

Salt and freshly ground black pepper, to taste ½ C. homemade vegetable broth

2 tsp. fresh lemon juice

For Rolls:

8 large cabbage leaves, rinsed 8 oz. sugar-free tomato sauce 3 tbsp. fresh basil leaves, chopped

Directions:

Preheat the oven to 400 0 F. Lightly, grease a 13x9-inch casserole dish.

For filling: in a large pan, add all the ingredients except the lemon juice over medium heat and bring to a boil.

Reduce the heat to low and simmer, covered for about 5 minutes.

Remove from the heat and set aside for about 5 minutes.

Add the lemon juice and stir to combine. Meanwhile, for rolls: in a large pan of the boiling water, add the cabbage leaves and boil for about 2-4 minutes. Drain the cabbage leaves well. Carefully, pat dry each cabbage leaf with paper towels.

Arrange the cabbage leaves onto a smooth surface.

With a knife, make a V shape cut in each leaf by cutting the thick vein.

Carefully, overlap cut ends of each leaf.

Place the filling mixture over each leaf evenly and fold in the sides.

Then, roll each leaf to seal the filling and then, secure each with toothpicks.

In the bottom of the prepared casserole dish, place 1/3 C. of the tomato sauce evenly.

Arrange the cabbage rolls over sauce in a single layer and top with remaining sauce evenly.

Cover the casserole dish and bake for about 15 minutes.

Remove from the oven and set aside, uncovered for about 5 minutes.

Serve warm with the garnishing of the basil.

Nutrition:

Calories: 33; Carbohydrates: 8.5g; Protein: 2.2g; Fat: 0.4g; Sugar: 4.3g;

Sodium: 225mg; Fiber: 1.9g

Chapter 16:

Desserts Recipes

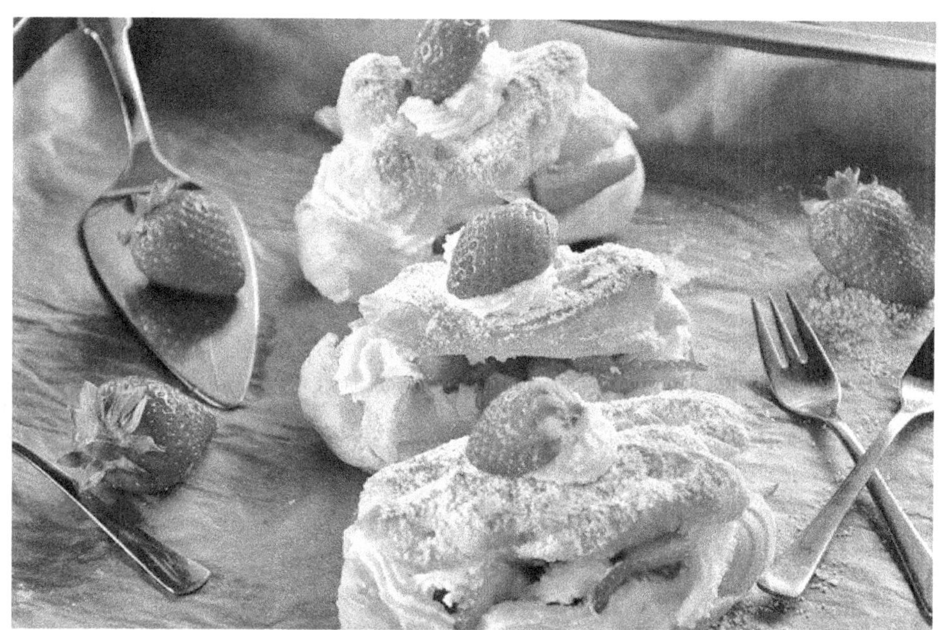

British Tartlets

Servings: 6

Cooking Time: 10 minutes

Preparation Time: 20 minutes

Ingredients:

For Crust: 2¼ C. almond flour ¼ C. powdered Swerve 5 tbsp. butter, melted ¼ tsp. sea salt

For Mascarpone Cream: 6 oz. mascarpone cheese, softened 2 tbsp. powdered Erythritol

1/3 C. heavy cream ¼ tsp. fresh lemon zest, grated 1 tsp. organic vanilla extract

For Garnishing: ½ C. fresh strawberries, hulled

Directions:

Preheat the oven to 350 0 F. Grease 6 (4-inch) tart pans. For crust: in a bowl, add all the ingredients and mix until well combined. Place the dough evenly into prepared tart pans and with your hands, press the mixture in the bottom and up sides. With a fork, prick the bottom of all crusts.

Bake for about 8-10 minutes.

Remove from the oven and place onto a wire rack to cool completely.

For the mascarpone cream: in a bowl, add mascarpone cheese, and Erythritol and with a mixer, beat on low speed for about 2 minutes. Slowly, add the heavy cream, beating continuously on low speed until well combined.

Now, beat on high speed for about 30-60 seconds or until thick. Add the lemon zest, and vanilla extract and beat until well combined.

Transfer the mascarpone cream into a piping bag, fitted with a large star shaped tip and fill the tartlets. Garnish with fresh strawberries and serve.

Nutrition:

Calories: 414; Carbohydrates: 10.8g; Protein: 12.5g;

Fat: 35.7g; Sugar: 0.6g; Sodium: 188mg; Fiber: 4.8g

Sweet & Tangy Tart

Servings: 12,

Cooking Time: 25 minutes,

Preparation Time: 20 minutes

Ingredients:

For Lemon Curd:

3 organic eggs 10 tbsp. powdered Erythritol 6 tbsp. fresh lemon juice

2 tsp. fresh lemon zest, grated 2 tbsp. butter

For Crust:

1½ C. blanched almond flour ½ C. coconut flour 4 tbsp. powdered Erythritol 2 organic eggs

4 tbsp. cold unsalted butter

For Topping:

12 oz. fresh raspberries

Directions:

For lemon curd: in a small non-stick pan, add the eggs, and Erythritol and beat until well combined. Now, add the lemon juice, and zest and beat until well combined. Place the pan over medium-low heat and cook for about 5-10 minutes or until mixture becomes thick, stirring continuously. Add the butter and stir until melted completely.

Remove from heat and transfer the curd into a bowl. With a cling film, cover the bowl and set aside for about 1 hour. Then, refrigerate for about 2 hours. Preheat the oven to 350 0 F. Line the bottom of 2 (9-inch) greased tart pans with a removable bottom. For crust: in a large bowl, add all the ingredients and mix until a dough ball comes together.

Divide the dough into 2 equal-sized portions.

Arrange 1 dough portion into each of the prepared tart pan and gently, press into the bottom to smooth the surface.

With a fork, prick the crust at many places.

Bake for about 15 minutes.

Remove the tart pans from oven and set aside to cool completely.

Gently and carefully, press each tart pan from the bottom to remove the sides.

Transfer each crust onto a platter.

Place the curd over each crust and with the back of a spoon, spread to smooth the surface.

Top each tart with fresh raspberries and serve.

Nutrition:

Calories: 198; Carbohydrates: 10.1g;

Protein: 6.5g; Fat: 15g;

Sugar: 1.6g; Sodium: 73mg; Fiber: 5.4g

Flour less Chocolate Cake

Servings: 8

Cooking Time: 15 minutes

Preparation Time: 28 minutes

Ingredients: 7 oz. 70% dark chocolate, chopped finely ½ C. olive oil 1 C. granulated Erythritol

5 large organic eggs 1 tsp. organic vanilla extract 4 tbsp. cacao powder 1 tsp. espresso powder

¼ tsp. salt

Directions:

Preheat the oven to 350 0 F. and lightly grease Line the bottom of a lightly greased 9-inch cake pan with parchment paper. In a microwave-safe bowl, add the chocolate and oil and microwave for about 2 minutes, stirring after every 30 seconds. Remove from the microwave and mix until smooth. Set aside to cool for about 2 of minutes. Add the Erythritol and beat until well combined. Add the eggs, one at a time, beating well after each addition. Add the vanilla extract and mix well. In another bowl, add the cocoa powder, espresso powder and salt and mix well. Add the cacao powder mixture into the chocolate mixture and mix until just combined. Place the mixture into the prepared cake pan evenly. Bake for about 25-28 minutes or until a skewer inserted in the center of comes out clean. Remove from the oven and place the pan onto a wire rack to cool for about 10-15 minutes. Carefully invert the cake and place onto the wire rack to cool completely before slicing. Cut into desired-sized slices and serve.

Nutrition: Calories: 326; Carbohydrates: 8.2g; Protein: 7.8g; Fat: 29.4g; Sugar: 0.3g;

Sodium: 126mg; Fiber: 4.1g

Melt-in-Moth Lava Cake

Servings: 2

Cooking Time: 9 minutes

Preparation Time: 15 minutes

Ingredients: 2 oz. 70% dark chocolate 2 oz. unsalted butter 2 organic eggs

2 tbsp. powdered Erythritol plus more for dusting 1 tbsp. almond flour 6 fresh raspberries

Directions:

Preheat the oven to 350 0 F. Grease 2 ramekins. In a microwave-safe bowl, add the chocolate and butter and microwave on High for about 2 minutes or until melted, stirring after every 30 seconds. Remove from the microwave and stir until smooth. Place the eggs in a bowl and with a wire whisk, beat well. Add the chocolate mixture, Erythritol and almond flour and mix until well combined. Divide the mixture into the prepared ramekins evenly. Bake for about 9 minutes or until the top is set. Remove from oven and set aside for about 1-2 minutes. Carefully, invert the cakes onto the serving plates and dust with extra powdered Erythritol. Serve with a garnishing of the strawberries.

Nutrition:

Calories: 436; Carbohydrates: 11g; Protein: 10.4g;

Fat: 25.2g; Sugar: 1.4g;

Sodium: 232mg; Fiber: 6.1g

British Tartlets

Servings: 6

Cooking Time: 10 minutes

Preparation Time: 20 minutes

Ingredients:

For Crust: 2¼ C. almond flour ¼ C. powdered Swerve 5 tbsp. butter, melted ¼ tsp. sea salt

For Mascarpone Cream: 6 oz. mascarpone cheese, softened 2 tbsp. powdered Erythritol

1/3 C. heavy cream ¼ tsp. fresh lemon zest, grated 1 tsp. organic vanilla extract

For Garnishing: ½ C. fresh strawberries, hulled

Directions: Preheat the oven to 350 0 F. Grease 6 (4-inch) tart pans. For crust: in a bowl, add all the ingredients and mix until well combined. Place the dough evenly into prepared tart pans and with your hands, press the mixture in the bottom and up sides. With a fork, prick the bottom of all crusts. Bake for about 8-10 minutes. Remove from the oven and place onto a wire rack to cool completely. For the mascarpone cream: in a bowl, add mascarpone cheese, and Erythritol and with a mixer, beat on low speed for about 2 minutes. Slowly, add the heavy cream, beating continuously on low speed until well combined. Now, beat on high speed for about 30-60 seconds or until thick. Add the lemon zest, and vanilla extract and beat until well combined. Transfer the mascarpone cream into a piping bag, fitted with a large star shaped tip and fill the tartlets. Garnish with fresh strawberries and serve.

Nutrition:Calories: 414; Carbohydrates: 10.8g; Protein: 12.5g; Fat: 35.7g; Sugar: 0.6g; Sodium: 188mg; Fiber: 4.8g

Sweet & Tangy Tart

Servings: 12

Cooking Time: 25 minutes

Preparation Time: 20 minutes

Ingredients:

For Lemon Curd: 3 organic eggs 10 tbsp. powdered Erythritol 6 tbsp. fresh lemon juice

2 tsp. fresh lemon zest, grated 2 tbsp. butter

For Crust: 1½ C. blanched almond flour ½ C. coconut flour 4 tbsp. powdered Erythritol

2 organic eggs 4 tbsp. cold unsalted butter

For Topping: 12 oz. fresh raspberries

Directions:

For lemon curd: in a small non-stick pan, add the eggs, and Erythritol and beat until well combined.

Now, add the lemon juice, and zest and beat until well combined.

Place the pan over medium-low heat and cook for about 5-10 minutes or until mixture becomes thick, stirring continuously.

Add the butter and stir until melted completely.

Remove from heat and transfer the curd into a bowl.

With a cling film, cover the bowl and set aside for about 1 hour.

Then, refrigerate for about 2 hours.

Preheat the oven to 350 0 F. Line the bottom of 2 (9-inch) greased tart pans with a removable bottom.

For crust: in a large bowl, add all the ingredients and mix until a dough ball comes together.

Divide the dough into 2 equal-sized portions.

Arrange 1 dough portion into each of the prepared tart pan and gently, press into the bottom to smooth the surface.

With a fork, prick the crust at many places.

Bake for about 15 minutes.

Remove the tart pans from oven and set aside to cool completely.

Gently and carefully, press each tart pan from the bottom to remove the sides.

Transfer each crust onto a platter.

Place the curd over each crust and with the back of a spoon, spread to smooth the surface.

Top each tart with fresh raspberries and serve.

Nutrition:

Calories: 198; Carbohydrates: 10.1g; Protein: 6.5g; Fat: 15g;

Sugar: 1.6g; Sodium: 73mg; Fiber: 5.4g

Light Greek Yogurt Cheesecake

Servings: 8

Cooking Time: 35 minutes

Preparation Time: 15 minutes

Ingredients: 2½ C. plain Greek yogurt 6-8 drops of liquid stevia 3 organic egg whites

1/3 C. cacao powder ¼ C. arrowroot starch 1 tsp. organic vanilla extract

Pinch of sea salt

Directions:

Preheat the oven to 35 0 F. Grease a 9-inch cake pan. In a large bowl, add all ingredients and mix until well combined. Place the mixture into the prepared pan evenly. Bake for about 30-35 minutes. Remove from oven and let it cool completely. Refrigerate to chill for about 3-4 hours or until set completely. Cut into 8 equal sized slices and serve.

Nutrition:

Calories: 85;

Carbohydrates: 10g; Protein: 6.4g;

Fat: 1.6g; Sugar: 5g;

Sodium: 97mg; Fiber: 2g

Swiss Roll Cake

Servings: 10

Cooking Time: 10 minutes

Preparation Time: 20 minutes

Ingredients:

For Cake:

1 C. almond flour ½ C. powdered Swerve ¼ C. matcha powder ¼ C. psyllium husk powder

1 tsp. organic baking powder ½ tsp. salt 3 large organic eggs

½ C. heavy whipping cream 4 tbsp. butter, melted 1 tsp. organic vanilla extract

For Filling:

3-4 tbsp. water 1 packet unflavored gelatin 2 C. heavy whipping cream

2 tsp. organic vanilla extract ¼ C. powdered Swerve

Directions:

Preheat oven to 350 0 F. Line a baking sheet with parchment paper.

For cake: in a bowl, add almond flour, Swerve, matcha powder, psyllium husk, baking powder and salt and mix well.

Now, sift the flour mixture into a second bowl.

In a third bowl, add remaining ingredients and beat until well combined.

Add the egg mixture into the bowl of flour mixture and mix until a very thick dough forms.

Place the dough onto prepared baking sheet and roll into an even rectangle.

Bake for about 10 minutes.

Remove from oven and put onto a wire rack to cool for about 4-5 minutes.

Gently, roll the warm cake with the help of parchment paper.

Set aside to cool completely.

For filling: in a microwave-safe bowl, add the water and sprinkle with the gelatin. Set aside for about 5 minutes.

 Now, microwave for about 15-20 seconds. Remove from microwave and beat the gelatin mixture until smooth.

Place gelatin mixture and remaining ingredients in bowl of the stand mixer and beat until cream becomes stiff. Spread the whipped cream over cooled cake evenly.

Carefully and gently, roll the cake and freezer for about 10 minutes before slicing.

Cut into desired sized slices and serve.

Nutrition:

Calories: 249; Carbohydrates: 7.1g; Protein: 5.6g; Fat: 22.8g;

Sugar: 0.7g; Sodium: 183mg; Fiber: 4g

Chapter 17:

Snacks Recipes

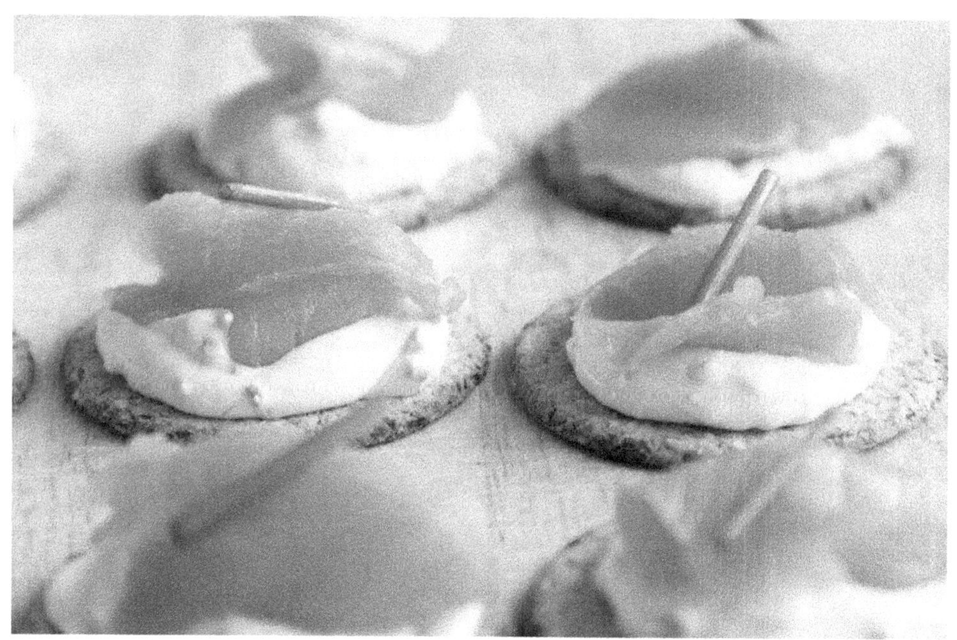

Crispy Broccoli Pop Corn

Preparation time: 15 minutes

Cooking time: 10 minutes

Servings: 4

Ingredients: 2 c. broccoli florets 2 c. coconut flour 4 egg yolks ½ tsp. salt ½ tsp. pepper

¼ c. butter

Directions:

Soak the broccoli florets in salty water to remove all the insects inside. Wash and rinse the broccoli florets then pat them dry.

Melt butter then let it cool. Crack the eggs then place in the same bowl with the melted butter.

Add coconut flour to the liquid then season with salt and pepper. Mix until incorporated.

Preheat an Air Fryer to 400°F (204°C).

Dip a broccoli floret in the coconut flour mixture then place in the Air Fryer. Repeat with the remaining broccoli florets.

Cook the broccoli florets 6 minutes. You may do this in several batches. Once it is done, remove the fried broccoli popcorn from the Air Fryer then place on a serving dish.

Serve and enjoy immediately.

Nutrition:

Calories: 202

Fat: 17.5g

Protein: 5.1g

Carbs: 7.8g

Cheesy Cauliflower Croquettes

Preparation time: 10 minutes

Cooking time: 16 minutes

Servings: 4

Ingredients:

2 c. cauliflower florets 2 tsps. minced garlic ½ c. chopped onion ¾ tsp. mustard

½ tsp. salt ½ tsp. pepper 2 tbsps. butter ¾ c. grated cheddar cheese

Directions:

Place butter in a microwave-safe bowl then melts the butter. Let it cool. Place cauliflower florets in a food processor then process until smooth and becoming crumbles. Transfer the cauliflower crumbles to a bowl then add chopped onion and cheese. Season with minced garlic, mustard, salt, and pepper then pour melted butter over the mixture. Shape the cauliflower mixture into medium balls then arrange in the Air Fryer.

Preheat an Air Fryer to 400°F (204°C) and cook the cauliflower croquettes for 14 minutes.

To achieve a more golden brown color, cook the cauliflower croquettes for another 2 minutes.

Serve and enjoy with homemade tomato sauce.

Nutrition:

Calories: 160 Fat: 13g Protein: 6.8g Carbs: 5.1g

Spinach in Cheese Envelopes

Preparation time: 15 minutes

Cooking time: 30 minutes

Servings: 8

Ingredients: 3 c. cream cheese 1½ c. coconut flour 3 egg yolks 2 eggs ½ c. cheddar cheese

2 c. steamed spinach ¼ tsp. salt ½ tsp. pepper ¼ c. chopped onion

Directions:

Place cream cheese in a mixing bowl then whisks until soft and fluffy. Add egg yolks to the mixing bowl then continue whisking until incorporated.

Stir in coconut flour to the cheese mixture then mix until becoming a soft dough. Place the dough on a flat surface then roll until thin. Cut the thin dough into 8 squares then keep. Crash the eggs then place in a bowl. Season with salt, pepper, and grated cheese then mix well. Add chopped spinach and onion to the egg mixture then stir until combined. Put spinach filling on a square dough then fold until becoming an envelope. Repeat with the remaining spinach filling and dough. Glue with water. Preheat an Air Fryer to 425°F (218°C). Arrange the spinach envelopes in the Air Fryer then cook for 12 minutes or until lightly golden brown.

Remove from the Air Fryer then serve warm. Enjoy!

Nutrition:

Calories: 365 Fat: 34.6g Protein: 10.4g Carbs: 4.4g

Cheesy Mushroom Slices

Preparation time: 8-10 minutes

Cooking time: 15 minutes

Servings: 8

Ingredients: 2 c. chopped mushrooms 2 eggs ¾ c. almond flour ½ c. grated cheddar cheese

2 tbsps. butter ½ tsp. pepper ¼ tsp. salt

Directions:

Place butter in a microwave-safe bowl then melts the butter.

Place chopped mushrooms in a food processor then add eggs, almond flour, and cheddar cheese.

Season with salt and pepper then pour melted butter into the food processor. Process until mixed. Transfer to a silicone loaf pan then spread evenly.

Preheat an Air Fryer to 375°F (191°C).

Place the loaf pan on the Air Fryer's rack then cook for 15 minutes. Once it is done, remove from the Air Fryer then let it cool.

Cut the mushroom loaf into slices then serve.

Enjoy!

Nutrition:

Calories: 365 Fat: 34.6g Protein: 10.4g Carbs: 4.4g

Asparagus Fries

Preparation time: 10 minutes

Cooking time: 10 minutes

Servings: 4

Ingredients: Medium organic asparagus spears – 10 Mayonnaise, full-fat – 3 tablespoon

Organic roasted red pepper, chopped – 1 tablespoon Almond flour – ¼ cup

Garlic powder – ½ teaspoon Smoked paprika – ½ teaspoon Chopped parsley – 2 tablespoons

Parmesan cheese, grated and full-fat – ½ cup Organic eggs, beaten – 2

Directions:

Set oven to 425 degrees F and preheat. Meanwhile, place cheese in a food processor, add garlic and parsley and pulse for 1 minute until fine mixture comes together. Add almond flour, pulse for 30 seconds until just mixed, then tip the mixture into a bowl and season with paprika. Crack eggs into a shallow dish and whisk until beaten. Working on one asparagus spear at a time, first dip into the egg mixture, then coat with parmesan mixture and place it on a baking sheet. Dip and coat more asparagus in the same manner, then arrange them on a baking sheet, 1-inch apart, and bake in the oven for 10 minutes or until asparagus is tender and nicely golden brown. Meanwhile, place mayonnaise in a bowl, add red pepper and whisk until combined and chill the dip into the refrigerator until required. Serve asparagus with prepared dip.

Nutrition:

Calories: 453 Fat: 33.4 g Protein: 19.1 g Net Carbs: 5.5 g Fiber: 3.75 g

Kale Chips

Preparation time: 5 minutes

Cooking time: 12 minutes

Servings: 4

Ingredients: Large bunch of organic kale – 1 Seasoned salt – 1 tablespoon

Olive oil – 2 tablespoons

Directions:

Set oven to 350 degrees F and preheat. Meanwhile, separate kale leaves from its stem, rinse the leaves under running water, then drain completely by using a vegetable spinner.

Wipe kale leaves with paper towels to remove excess water, then transfer them into a large plastic bag and add oil.

Seal the plastic bag, turn it upside down until kale is coated with oil and then spread kale leaves on a large baking sheet.

Place the baking sheet into the oven and bake for 12 minutes or until its edges are nicely golden brown.

Remove baking sheet from the oven, season kale with salt and serve.

Nutrition:

Calories: 163 Fat: 10 g Protein: 2 g Net Carbs: 14 g Fiber: 2 g

Guacamole

Preparation time: 10 minutes

Cooking time: 0 minutes

Servings: 4

Ingredients:

Organic avocados, pitted – 2 Medium organic red onion, peeled and sliced – 1/3

Medium organic jalapeño, deseeded and diced – 1 Salt – ½ teaspoon

Ground pepper – ½ teaspoon Tomato salsa, organic – 2 tablespoons

Lime juice, organic – 1 tablespoon Bunch of organic cilantro – ½

Directions:

Cut each avocado into half, remove its pit and slice its flesh horizontally and vertically.

Scoop out the flesh of the avocado, place it in a bowl and add onion, jalapeno, and lime juice then stir until well mixed.

Season with salt and black pepper, add salsa and stir with a fork until avocado is mash to desired consistency.

Fold in cilantro and serve.

Nutrition:

Calories: 16.5 Fat: 1.4 g Protein: 0.23 g Net Carbs: 0.5 g Fiber: 0.6 g

Zucchini Noodles

Preparation time: 5 minutes

Cooking time: 6 minutes

Servings: 2

Ingredients: Medium zucchini, spiralized into noodles – 2 Butter, unsalted – 2 tablespoons

Minced garlic – 1 ½ tablespoon Parmesan cheese, grated – 3/4 cup Sea salt – ½ teaspoon

Ground black pepper – ¼ teaspoon Red chili flakes – ¼ teaspoon

Directions:

Switch on the instant pot, add butter, press the 'sauté/simmer' button, wait until the butter melts, and add garlic and cook for 1 minute or until fragrant.

Add zucchini noodles, toss until coated, cook for 5 minutes or until tender and season with salt and black pepper.

Press the 'keep warm' button, then transfer to noodles to a dish, top with cheese and sprinkle with red chili flakes.

Serve straight away.

Nutrition:

Calories: 298 Fat: 26.1 g Protein: 5 g Net Carbs: 2.3 g Fiber: 0.1 g

Cauliflower Souffle

Preparation time: 10 minutes

Cooking time: 12 minutes

Servings: 6

Ingredients: Large head of Cauliflower, cut into small florets – 1 Eggs – 2

Heavy Cream – 2 tablespoons Cream Cheese – 2 ounces Sour Cream – 1/2 cup

Asiago cheese – 1/2 cup Sharp Cheddar Cheese, grated – 1 cup Chives – ¼ cup

Butter, unsalted – 2 tablespoons slices of bacon, sugar-free, cooked, crumbled – 6 Water – 1 cup

Directions:

Crack eggs in a food processor, add heavy cream, sour cream, cream cheese, and cheeses and pulse until smooth. Add cauliflower florets, pulse for 2 seconds or until folded and chunky, then add butter and chives and pulse for another 2 seconds. Switch on the instant pot, pour in water, and insert a trivet stand. Pour the cauliflower mixture in a greased round casserole dish that fits into the instant pot, smooth the top and place the dish on the trivet stand. Shut the instant pot with its lid in the sealed position, then press the 'manual' button, press '+/-' to set the cooking time to 12 minutes and cook at high-pressure setting; when the pressure builds in the pot, the cooking timer will start. When the instant pot buzzes, press the 'keep warm' button, release pressure naturally for 10 minutes, then do a quick pressure release and open the lid. Take out the casserole dish, top with bacon, and serve.

Nutrition:

Calories: 342 Fat: 28 g Protein: 17 g Net Carbs: 5 g Fiber: 2 g

Chapter 18:

Tips On Losing Weight On Keto After 50

In this chapter, I will go over a few more things you can do so you can optimize your weight loss.

<u>Exercise</u>

In the fitness world, it is already established that 80% of your weight loss success comes from the diet. So just by following the keto diet alone, you are already making great progress. However, if you want that extra edge in your weight loss, consider doing exercises.

You have plenty of options here. You can do cardio exercises such as jogging, running or cycling every morning for 30 minutes, but strength training works just as well for older adults. In fact, you should do both if you can.

Cardio exercises can get the heart pumping and get the body moving more freely, but note that your muscle mass starts to decline after 50. So work on your muscles as well.

How much exercise should you do? It depends on how much you can handle. No point in pushing beyond the limit and regret it later, right?

<u>Team Up</u>

A group activity is always more entertaining. So if you can find like-minded individuals who are also into keto diets, consider doing it together with them. It makes things much easier. This tip also applies to some other tips that I will show you, such as exercise that I just covered.

Move More

Moving more here does not mean more cardio exercises. You cannot expect to get any more effective weight loss if you exercise for 30mns a day and then sit on the couch for the rest of the day. The idea is to burn more calories than you can take in, so it pays to be a little extra active throughout the day.

If you have a desk job, consider getting up at least once an hour and take a short break by walking in the lobby for at least 5 minutes. It doesn't seem much, but it helps in the long run.

More Protein

Protein is very important for both weight loss and youth, including the protection against muscle degradation and other aging ailments. Couple a high protein intake with strength exercise and you can be sure that you would be building muscles faster than they can degrade. You won't look like Arnold when he was a bodybuilder, but you might even look fitter than the guy in his 20s at your workplace.

Talk to a Dietitian

The first thing you should do before getting into any diet is to consult your dietitian. While the keto diet works for many people, you never really know if it will work for you. Therefore, it is wise to ask your dietitian first before you jump in, rather than suffer some adverse effects because your body is not compatible with this diet.

Cook at Home More

Or eat out less frequently. There are two reasons why you should do that. For one, there are only a few places, if at all, that serve keto-based foods, let alone those that follow your diet plan. You need to prepare your own food if you want to do a keto diet. Another benefit is economics. You will buy most of your ingredients and prepare your meals ahead of time. This means you will only spend your money on the ingredients you know you will need.

Eat More Produce

While we are on the subject of eating, consider incorporating more produces in your diet, some of which I have covered already. Vegetables and fruits are full of nutrients that your body needs to remain healthy, so it should be included in your diet.

Hire a Personal Trainer

While we are still discussing exercising, consider getting yourself a personal trainer. That way, you can get the most out of your exercises and your trainer also doubles as an exercise partner as well because they hold you accountable for your own commitments. Your trainer is very helpful when you do strength training because they can teach you how to perform the exercise with the correct form and preventing you from injuring yourself.

Rely Less on Convenience Foods

Convenient foods are convenient, but not healthy. Not by a long shot. They are rich in calories and often do not pack essential nutrients such as protein, fiber, vitamins, etc. If you can, ditch convenient foods altogether.

Find an Activity You Enjoy

When you have done enough exercise, you will know what activities you like. One way to encourage yourself to exercise more regularly is by making it entertaining than a chore. If possible, stick to your favorite activities and you can get the most out of your exercises. Keep in mind that the activities you enjoy may not be effective or needed, so you need to find other exercises to compensate, which you may not enjoy so much. For instance, if you like jogging, then you can really work your leg muscles, but your arms are not involved. So you need to do pushups or other strength training exercises.

Here, your trainer can help you decide and create a workout routine that you can stick with as well.

Check with a Healthcare Provider

As mentioned earlier, the keto diet works for many people, but it isn't for everyone. Your dietitian can tell you whether keto diet would work, but it helps to check in with your healthcare provider to ensure that you do not have any medical condition that prevents you from losing weight, such as hypothyroidism and polycystic ovarian syndrome. It helps to know well in advance whether your body is even capable of losing fat in the first place before you commit and see no result, right?

Eat Less at Night

While the science still argues about it to this day, it seems more logical that breakfast is the most important meal of the day considering that you would not have eaten for the past 8 hours whereas the interval between breakfast and lunch, and lunch and dinner is 5 or 6 hours at best. By the same token, dinner should be small because your body does not need to expend that much energy when you are sleeping anyway. So the excess energy becomes fat.

So keep dinner light. For one, it helps you lose weight. Another reason is if you have a heavy dinner, your body will strain itself trying to digest everything. That means your body would remain active until all the food is digested, meaning that you will not get restful sleep if you can sleep at all.

Bottom line: Eat light and eat dinner at least 4 hours prior to bedtime. Any sooner and you will have a hard time sleeping.

Body Composition

Your body isn't just "weight" alone. Your body is composed of fat, muscles, fluid, bones, etc. What you want to lose is fat weight, not muscle weight or fluid weight. You want as little fat mass in your body as possible while still maintaining a healthy level of non-fat mass in your body. There are many ways you can measure your body fat, but the simplest method is to measure your calves, thighs, waist, chest, and biceps.

Hydrate Properly

That means drinking enough water or herbal tea and ditch sweetened beverages or other drinks that contain sugar altogether. Making the transition will be difficult for the first few weeks, but your body will be thanking you for it. There is nothing healthier than good old plain water and the recommended amount is 2 gallons a day. However, because you are on a keto diet, your body needs to use up more water so consider 2 gallons to the absolute minimum amount of water you need to drinks. I recommend you drink between 3 or even 4 gallons a day when you are on a keto diet. If you get thirsty, then it is a sign of dehydration, so drink some water. Drinking plenty of water also leads to additional calories burned. You can shave off a few more calories by drinking cold water because your body will spend more energy trying to regulate your body temperature.

Supplements

When you get older, your body starts to lose its ability to absorb certain nutrients, which leads to deficits. For example, vitamin B12 and folate are some of the most common nutrients that people over 50 lack. They have an impact on your mood, energy level, and weight loss rate.

Therefore, if you feel tired when you are on your keto diet, perhaps you do not get enough nutrients that your body needs. That does not mean you should eat more, no. You just need to take the right supplements.

Get Enough Sleep

When you are over 50, your body starts to fail you. You no longer have the ability to party past midnight without feeling horrible for the rest of the month. If there is the most crucial time to get 8 hours of sleep a day, then it is right now.

Getting enough sleep helps your body regulate the hormones in your body, so try to aim for 7 to 9 hours of sleep a day. You can get more restful sleep by creating a nighttime routine that involves not looking at a computer, phone, or TV screen for at least 1 hour before bed. You can drink warm milk or water to help your body relax, or even do 10 to 20 minutes of stretching so you can get a restful sleep.

While we are on the subject of sleeping, try to maintain a consistent sleeping schedule. I understand that you want to sleep and wake up 1 to 4 hours later than usual during the weekend. But you want to go to bed and wake up at the same time, your mood and energy level will be higher. An added benefit is that your body will learn to wake up on its own even without the alarm.

Mindful Eating

Mindfulness isn't restricted to meditation alone. Again, we will not go over meditation in this book because it is another topic altogether. But what you can do here is learn to love and appreciate your food. It sounds obnoxious, but it helps your mood and promotes weight loss.

Simply put, you just have to put away your phone and take away any other sources of distractions and focus solely on your food, how it tastes, etc. That means eating slowly. You will learn to appreciate how tasty your food is because you actually focus on eating.

How does this translate to weight loss? You see, there is a system in your body that determines how full you are. The issue here is that this system is not instantaneous. It takes some time to measure how full your stomach it before sending the signal to your brain. So when you eat too quickly, by the time you feel full, you would have already overshot by a country mile. If you eat slowly, your body has enough time to register your fullness bite by bite. So when you feel full, you have not overeaten.

<u>Use Inconvenience to Your Advantage</u>

The problem is that just ditching these delicious snacks cold turkey style is difficult, especially if you have developed a taste for them. So what do you do? Well, you remove such food from your house immediately. Only have enough food in the house for the week or have only healthy snacks in the house.

Even when you have a sudden craving for unhealthy snacks, the inconvenience of going out to buy one is enough to dissuade you and help you suppress the hunger. Another solution is to tell yourself that you will grab that unhealthy snack "tomorrow". We are all professional procrastinators or were one at a certain point in our lives, so use that to your advantage as well. When you set a "plan" like that, your mind is tricked into thinking that you will get around to it when the time is right, although that time will never come.

But what if you need to go out and get groceries for next week's keto meals? You have two options.

You can go to the grocery store carrying just enough money to get everything you need for next week's meals. That way, you simply cannot afford to buy extra snacks. But this requires your prior knowledge of the prices of the products you need to buy, and any price changes can leave you with some extra change or you not having enough money. To remedy this problem, I recommend you bring a bit extra just in case there are any price changes.

An alternative that I like is to bring someone along with you for the trip, but you let them carry all the money. The amount does not matter here, but it requires the other person to be firm about not letting you buy that potato chip. They have the money and they will have to stick to the plan of buying enough for the week, nothing more than that. It is going to be a bit inconvenient for the other person, but they can hold you accountable and keep you in control of the situation.

Conclusion

Keto diet provides long term health benefits compare to other diet plans. During keto diet near about 75 to 90 percent of calories comes from fats, an adequate number of calories 5 to 20 percent comes from proteins and 5 percent of calories from carb intake.

What began as a simple spark of curiosity ended on a high note: keto, a term you constantly read and heard about. Now you have all the knowledge in the world to lead a lifestyle that is truly worthy of your time, energy, and effort.

Being 50 years old or more is not bad. It is how we handle ourselves in this age that matters. Most of us would have just moved on and dealt with things as they would have arrived. That is no longer the case. It is quite literally survival of the fittest.

With keto, you are among the fittest people in existence. Your lifestyle will change dramatically but it would be quite a pleasant change; one that you can be proud of.

Do not give up now as there will be quite a few days where you may think to yourself, "Why am I doing this?" and to answer that, simply focus on the goals you wish to achieve.

Whether you wish to stay active, lose weight, look and feel better, or any of that, keto is your solution and a way of life that will ensure you get all that you need.

A good diet enriched with all the proper nutrients is our best shot of achieving an active metabolism and efficient lifestyle. A lot of people think that the Keto diet is simply for people who are interested in losing weight. You will find that it is quite the opposite. There are intense keto diets where only 5 percent of the diet comes from carbs, 20 percent is from protein, and 75 percent is from fat. But even a modified version of this which involves consciously choosing foods low in carbohydrate and high in healthy fats is good enough.

Thanks for reading this book. I hope it has provided you with enough insight to get you going. Don't put off getting started. The sooner you begin this diet, the sooner you'll start to notice an improvement in your health and well-being.